Disclaimer: the inforr

educational purposes only, and does not substitute for professional medical advice.

To request permission contact the publisher at goodlookinbooks@gmail.com

Softcover ISBN: 979-8-9865663-3-7

References: TNoncology.com and The American Cancer Society

The GoodLook In Books Corp.
www.thegoodlookinbooks.com

Dedication:

To the woman who is dealing with the pain, the awkwardness, the annoyance of trying on clothes, the uncomfortable gestures made by others. This is for YOU. This will be the time where you get through this and start to feel like a new person. You never know what will transpire in your life at the time of this surgery, so keep that in mind. During this time you could be going through a break up, your menstrual cycle (where you are super emotional), you could be grieving or going through financial hardships. Be prepared to go through it before you get through it. Believe in your power to heal, to become stronger and more vibrant than you were before. I believe in your strength, your courage and your power to becoming and embracing the new YOU.

Second I am going to dedicate this to the man who is constantly looking at her breasts instead of her eyes. The man who will always talk about how big your breasts are but never gives you a compliment on how beautiful you are inside and out. I dedicated this to you because besides the daily uncomforting moments we feel with the pain in our back, shoulders and clothes, you make us feel extra uncomfortable with these actions. So if this book comes across your hands I encourage you, to encourage your woman with softness and appreciation for who she is vs what she carries on her chest.

Introduction:

I created this guided journal because during my breast reduction recovery I felt alone. I wanted to hear people give some encouraging words, I needed support but without telling the world what I was feeling and it just seemed as if there was nothing available all in one easy access. I am not sure if people know that this recovery process is just that a process, not a race. So I did this for you, the next woman who will be going through the same.

Even if you have help, you are the only one going through these changes. This surgery is emotionally, physically and mentally challenging. So, I came up with this journal to give you some exercise routines, positive words, motivation and some extra tips on what to do to feel better. Keep in mind that the healing process of any procedure or life changing event can vary from person to person.

However, I can assure you that if you take the necessary steps in keeping a strong mindset throughout the process your journey would be so much more easier and worth it all. I want to emphasize that when I say keep a strong mindset I don't mean you can't cry or feel discouraged or feel the pain, I want you to go through everything. However most importantly I want you to GROW through everything. So here is my guided book on helping YOU embrace the new YOU.

Here are some tips that helped me through out my breast reduction healing journey.

In the first few days you are unable to bathe but I did get in the shower and use a cup to pour the water over my body to rinse off.

When the doctors give you permission to bathe, buy yourself a long handle washing loofah brush. Even with that it still may be difficult to get to certain areas but it is helpful having it rather than not.

Turn your back to the water do not let it run on your breast until you are told by your physician. Even then I personally still waited some time. I did not feel comfortable with the water touching my breasts. Use your discretion.

I recommend you use a blow dryer to dry under your breast on the incision.
You won't be able to dry with a towel for some time, so to avoid infection that area must be dry.

When you are able to take off your bandages you will not see your breasts in the ending result. They will look swollen, they will obviously look different and it can cause shock or complete joy.

Take it in gradually, if you cry it is ok too, I surely did but, I eventually came to a better headspace once I started to do the steps in this book. Remember this is a process and it is going to take time.

You will have to start massaging your breasts at some point to help smooth out lumps that occur from your surgery. I recommend you get yourself a breast massager and use warm compresses. It was a great investment and I massaged my breasts daily for months. In addition to adding herbal creams which were also amazing for the burning sensation that happens as well. Even with me taking care of myself I still ended up with a hematoma. (*A pool of mostly clotted blood that forms in an organ, tissue, or body space.*)

However, I know that it was meant for me to be still. Which is something else I want to elaborate on.

Take your time and do not rush to go out, or do anything that will prolong your healing. I know that some women may not have any assistance and we may have no choice to do certain things and that is understandable but do not rush to go out to party or be social. Your body needs time and nourishment and so does your mind and spirit and you do not want to do anything to break that.

A breast reduction is a major surgery and you will not be able to do half of the things you were able to prior. However with eating right, Drinking lots of water. taking your herbs/meds, exercising at your pace and meditating you will be able to get into a good space. Be sure to get yourself some compression bras and don't be afraid to spend the money, you will need good quality bras for support.

Meals are a very important part of the healing process. It is vital that you avoid foods that are harmful to your body. You need to help build your cells back up.

My suggestion is to fast, juicing which would consist of veggies and or fruits, avoid sugar and anything fried or fatty. Even take the time to eliminate dairy and meats from your diet and find some good herbal supplements to help the process.

I took bromelain, Seamoss with other herbs such as soursop, bladderwrack, burdock root, moringa and more. Herbal teas instead of coffee. Yarrow is really good for wound healing and inflammation.

To add I highly recommended a few different pillows, the first is a breast pillow which will help protect you while in a vehicle or outside. They come with pockets to keep your phone, remote or anything you need easy access to. The others are a pregnancy pillow to help secure you while lying down and extras on the bed to keep you tucked and secure.

Meditation is a great way to help with any shock, depression, uncertainty, mental clarity and just overall daily life.
There are many people who do not know how to meditate so I encourage you to look up some guided meditation videos to help you through. You can also put some meditation music, breathe in through your nose and out through your mouth and say mantras that will help you get through the days. I gave an example of three mantras that you can repeat but please say whatever feels better for your spirit.

Look out the window and let the sun hit you directly, close your eyes and breathe. This is also a good time to get those arms of yours to move. I know they are feeling stiff and you are probably hunch over from the awkwardness feeling you have from surgery. Next I am going to give you some examples of exercises that helped me.

The tips and exercises listed below should be done for the first 3 to 7 days after surgery. Do not do them until you get the OK from your doctor

Practice deep breathing exercises (using your diaphragm) at least 6 times a day. Lie down on your back and take a slow, deep breath. Breathe in as much air as you can while trying to expand your chest and abdomen (push your belly button away from your spine). Relax and breathe out. Repeat this 4 or 5 times. This exercise will help maintain normal movement of your chest, making it easier for your lungs to work. Do deep breathing exercises often.

Do the exercises slowly until you feel a gentle stretch. Hold each stretch at the end of the motion and slowly count to 5. It's normal to feel some pulling as you stretch the skin and muscles that have been shortened because of the surgery. You should not feel pain as you do them, only gentle stretching.

Do each exercise 5 to 7 times. Try to do each exercise correctly. If you have trouble with the exercises, talk to your doctor. You may need to be referred to a physical or occupational therapist.

Do the exercises twice a day until you get back your normal flexibility.

Be sure to take deep breaths, in and out, as you do each exercise.

The exercises are set up so that you start them lying down, move to sitting, and finish them standing up.

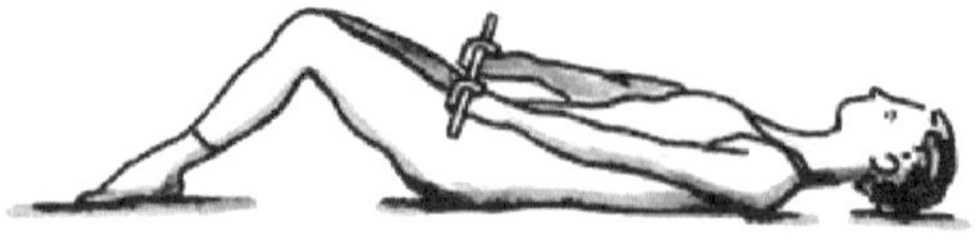

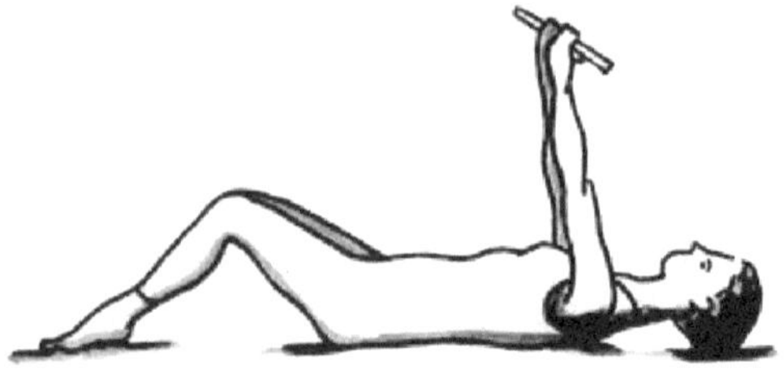

This exercise also helps increase shoulder blade movement.

Sit in a chair in front of a mirror. Face straight ahead. Do not rest against the back of the chair.
Your arms should be at your sides with your elbows bent.
Squeeze your shoulder blades together, bringing your elbows behind you. Keep your shoulders level as you do this. Do not lift your shoulders up toward your ears.
Return to the starting position and repeat 5 to 7 times.

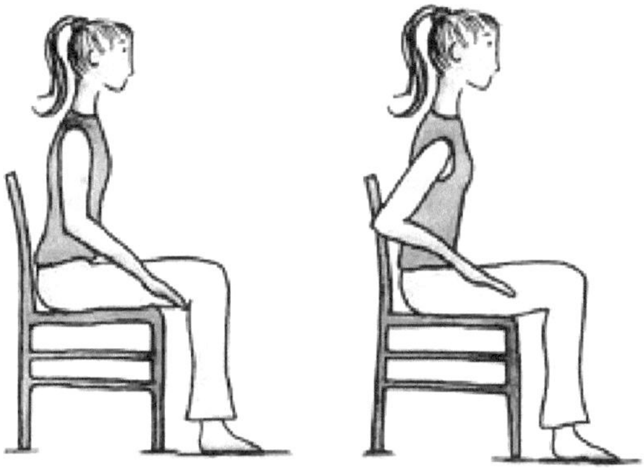

This exercise helps increase movement of your trunk and body.

Sit in a chair and clasp your hands together in front of you. Lift your arms slowly over your head, straightening your arms.
When your arms are over your head, bend your trunk to the right keeping your arms overhead.
Return to the starting position and bend to the left.
Repeat 5 to 7 times.

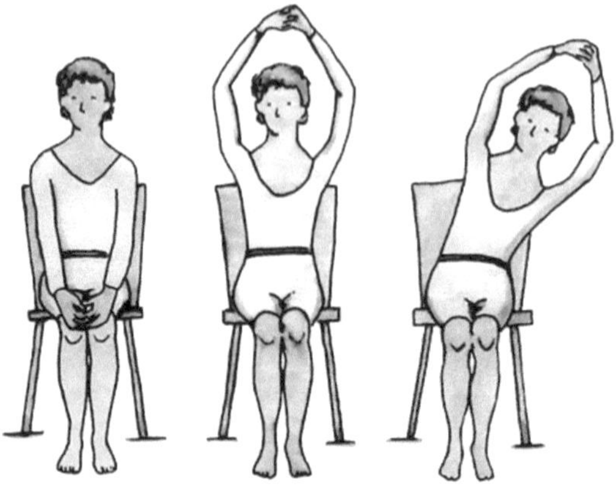

This exercise helps increase your mobility in your shoulder.

Stand facing the wall with your toes about 8 to 10 inches from the wall.
Put your hands on the wall. Use your fingers to “climb the wall,” reaching as high as you can until you feel a stretch.
Return to the starting position and repeat 5 to 7 times.
The picture shows both arms going up at the same time, but you might find it easier to raise one arm at a time.
Be sure you keep your shoulders dropped far away from your ears as you raise your arms.
This will happen within time, throughout your 90 days you will see your arms reaching higher.

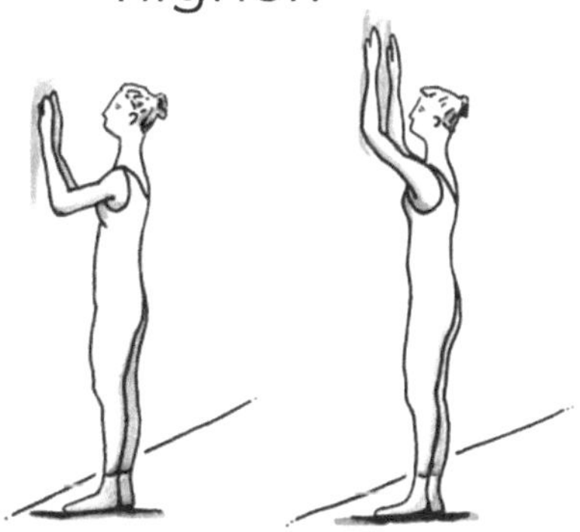

Things to keep in mind after breast surgery
Start exercising slowly and increase as you are able. Stop exercising and talk to your doctor right away if you:

Get weaker, start losing your balance, or start falling
Have pain that gets worse
Have new heaviness, aching, tightness, or other strange sensations in your arm
Have unusual swelling or swelling gets worse
Have headaches, dizziness, blurred vision, new numbness, or tingling in your arms or chest
It's important to exercise to keep your muscles working as well as possible, but it's also important to be safe. Talk with your doctor about the right kind of exercises for your condition, and then set goals for increasing your level of physical activity.

Start Your Day with These 5 M's...

MEDITATION

CLOSE EYES, BREATHE, FOCUS ON GETTING THROUGH THE PAIN AND THE PROCESS. PUT ON MEDITATION MUSIC IF IT HELPS.

MEDICATIONS:

TAKE YOUR HERBS AND/OR MEDICATIONS. DEPENDING ON YOUR LIFESTYLE.

IF THE PAIN PILLS MAKE YOU FEEL SICK FIND ALTERNATIVES TO HELP WITH PAIN.

MOVEMENTS:

MOVING YOUR BODY WILL HELP HEAL FASTER. I KNOW IT IS DIFFICULT BUT YOU HAVE TO MAKE AN EFFORT IN STARTING WITH WALKING AROUND YOUR HOME FOR 15 MINUTES TO START FOR THE 1ST WEEK EVERY DAY TWICE A WEEK. FOLLOW THE IMAGES AND INFO FOR EXERCISES IN BEGINNING OF THE BOOK TO HELP START MOVEMENT IN YOUR UPPER BODY

MANTRAS:

I AM STRONGER THAN I KNOW

I WILL HEAL AT PEACE AND AT MY OWN PACE.

I WILL GET BETTER AND BETTER EACH DAY

MEALS

IT IS IMPORTANT TO EAT FOOD HIGH IN VITAMIINS AND NUTRIENTS.
AVOID FAST FOODS, MEATS AND FRIED ANYTHING.
YOUR BODY IS GOING THROUGH A MAJOR SHOCK AND EVERYTHING THAT YOU DO GOING FORWARD WILL IMPACT THE PROCESS OF YOUR HEALING. JUICING AND FASTING CAN HELP YOU AS WELL. MAKE SURE TO DRINK LOTS OF WATER!

LETS GO THROUGH THE CHECKLIST DAY 1

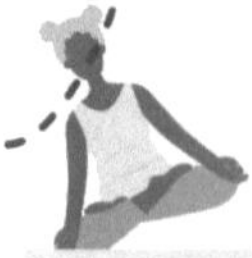

DID YOU MEDITATE?

HOW LONG?

HOW DO YOU FEEL?

DID YOU MAKE SURE TO BREATHE?

DON'T FORGET YOUR MANTRAS.

MEDS AND HERBS INTAKE

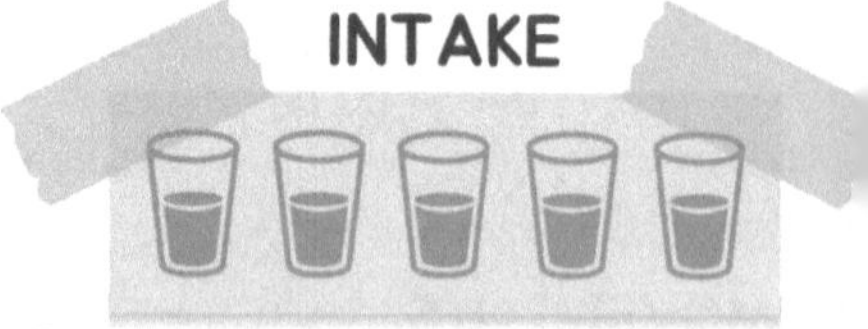

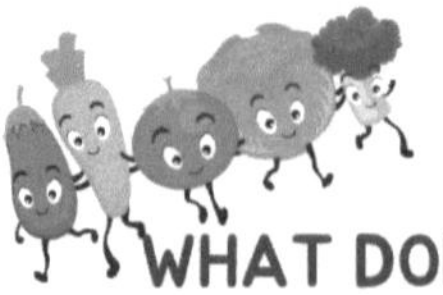

WHAT DOES YOUR MEAL LOOK LIKE TODAY

Breakfast:

Lunch:

Dinner:

Snack:

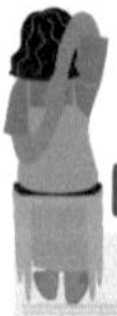

HOW WERE YOUR MOVEMENTS TODAY?

LETS GO THROUGH THE CHECKLIST DAY 2

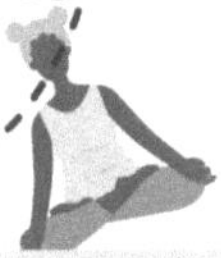

DID YOU MEDITATE?

HOW LONG?

HOW DO YOU FEEL?

DID YOU MAKE SURE TO BREATHE?

DON'T FORGET YOUR MANTRAS.

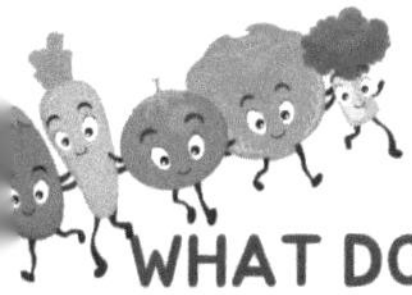

WHAT DOES YOUR MEAL LOOK LIKE TODAY

Breakfast:

Lunch:

Dinner:

Snack:

MEDS AND HERBS INTAKE

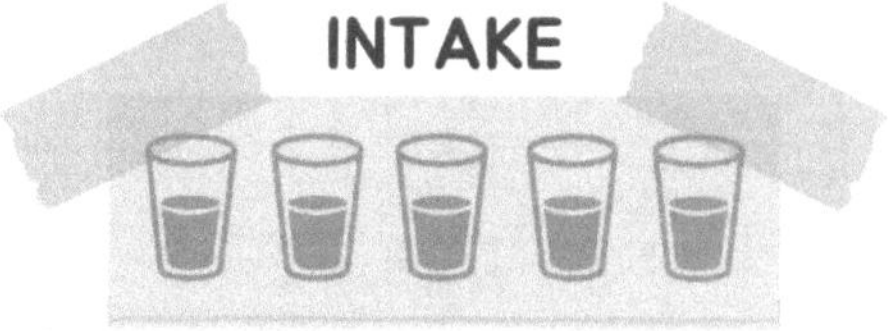

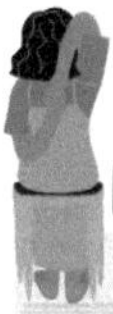

HOW WERE YOUR MOVEMENTS TODAY?

LETS GO THROUGH THE CHECKLIST DAY 3

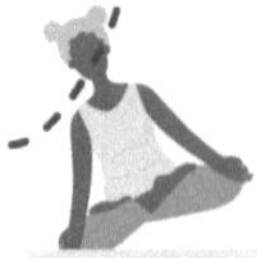

DID YOU MEDITATE?

HOW LONG?

HOW DO YOU FEEL?

DID YOU MAKE SURE TO BREATHE?

DON'T FORGET YOUR MANTRAS.

MEDS AND HERBS INTAKE

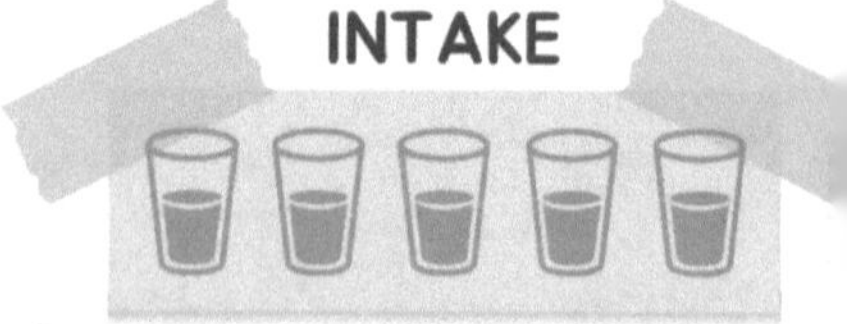

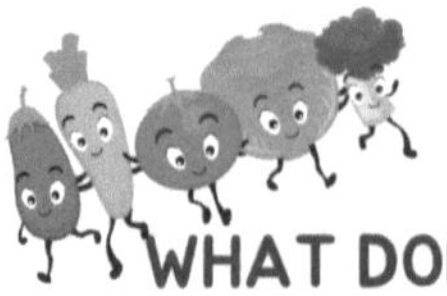

WHAT DOES YOUR MEAL LOOK LIKE TODAY

Breakfast:

Lunch:

Dinner:

Snack:

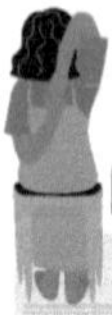

HOW WERE YOUR MOVEMENTS TODAY?

LETS GO THROUGH THE CHECKLIST DAY 4

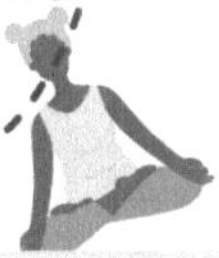

DID YOU MEDITATE?

HOW LONG?

HOW DO YOU FEEL?

DID YOU MAKE SURE TO BREATHE?

DON'T FORGET YOUR MANTRAS.

MEDS AND HERBS INTAKE

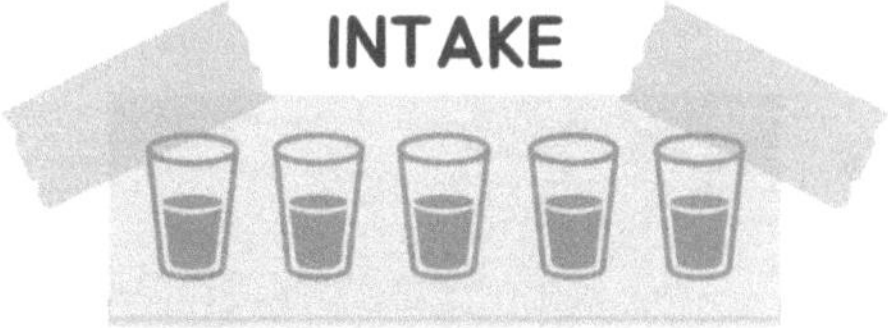

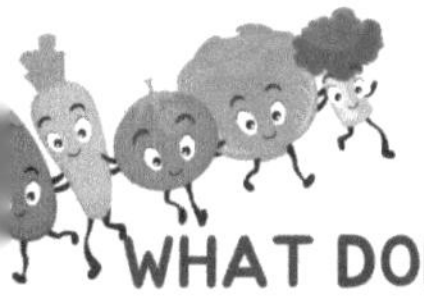

WHAT DOES YOUR MEAL LOOK LIKE TODAY

Breakfast:

Lunch:

Dinner:

Snack:

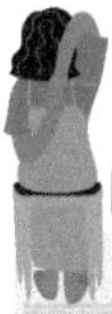

HOW WERE YOUR MOVEMENTS TODAY?

LETS GO THROUGH THE CHECKLIST DAY 5

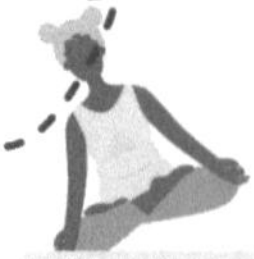

DID YOU MEDITATE?

HOW LONG?

HOW DO YOU FEEL?

DID YOU MAKE SURE TO BREATHE?

DON'T FORGET YOUR MANTRAS.

MEDS AND HERBS INTAKE

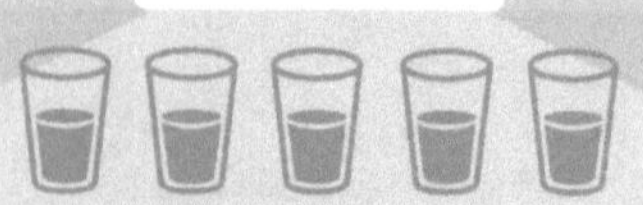

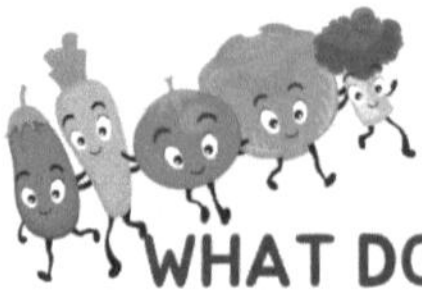

WHAT DOES YOUR MEAL LOOK LIKE TODAY

Breakfast:

Lunch:

Dinner:

Snack:

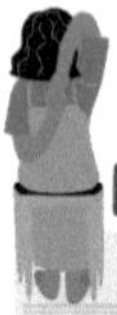

HOW WERE YOUR MOVEMENTS TODAY?

LETS GO THROUGH THE CHECKLIST DAY 6

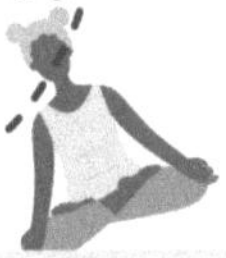

DID YOU MEDITATE?

HOW LONG?

HOW DO YOU FEEL?

DID YOU MAKE SURE TO BREATHE?

DON'T FORGET YOUR MANTRAS.

MEDS AND HERBS INTAKE

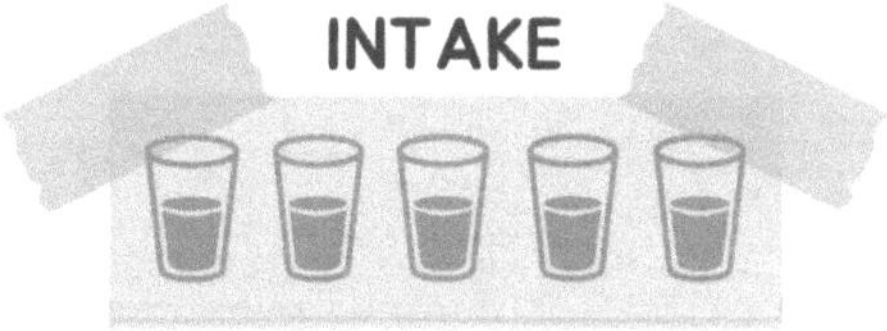

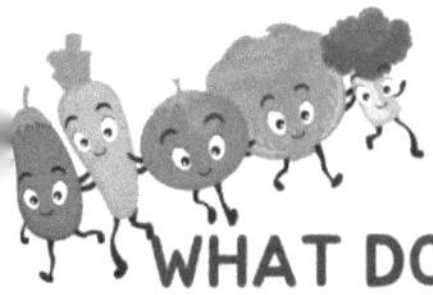

WHAT DOES YOUR MEAL LOOK LIKE TODAY

Breakfast:

Lunch:

Dinner:

Snack:

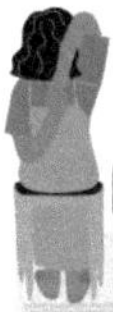

HOW WERE YOUR MOVEMENTS TODAY?

LETS GO THROUGH THE CHECKLIST DAY 7

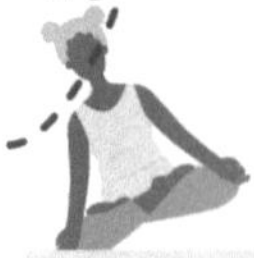

DID YOU MEDITATE?

HOW LONG?

HOW DO YOU FEEL?

DID YOU MAKE SURE TO BREATHE?

DON'T FORGET YOUR MANTRAS.

MEDS AND HERBS INTAKE

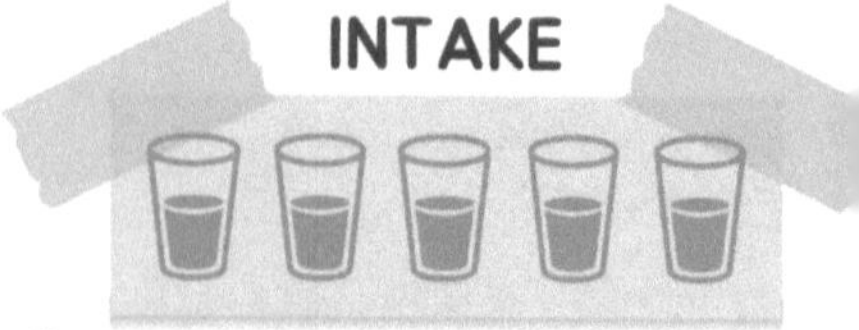

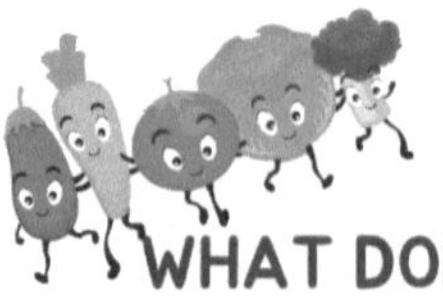

WHAT DOES YOUR MEAL LOOK LIKE TODAY

Breakfast:

Lunch:

Dinner:

Snack:

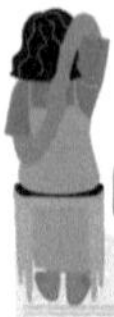

HOW WERE YOUR MOVEMENTS TODAY?

KEEP PUSHING
YOU ARE YOUR
THOUGHTS!
WHAT YOU THINK
WILL BE YOUR
ENDING RESULTS.
SO THINK POSITIVE!

LETS GO THROUGH THE CHECKLIST DAY 8

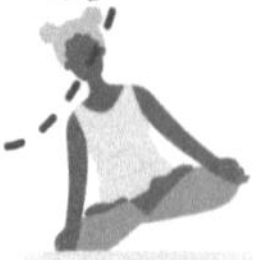

DID YOU MEDITATE?

HOW LONG?

HOW DO YOU FEEL?

DID YOU MAKE SURE TO BREATHE?

DON'T FORGET YOUR MANTRAS.

MEDS AND HERBS INTAKE

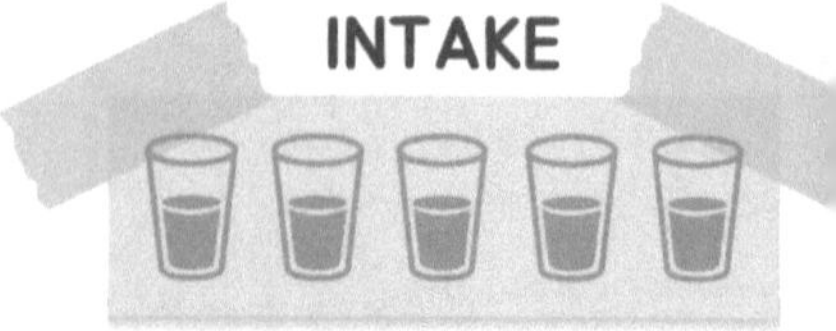

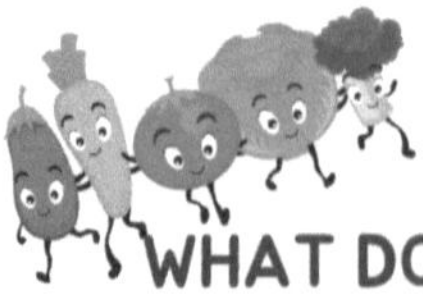

WHAT DOES YOUR MEAL LOOK LIKE TODAY

Breakfast:

Lunch:

Dinner:

Snack:

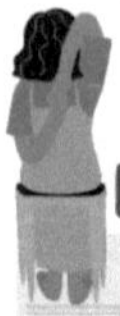

HOW WERE YOUR MOVEMENTS TODAY?

LETS GO THROUGH THE CHECKLIST DAY 9

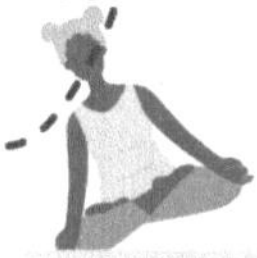

DID YOU MEDITATE?

HOW LONG?

HOW DO YOU FEEL?

DID YOU MAKE SURE TO BREATHE?

DON'T FORGET YOUR MANTRAS.

MEDS AND HERBS INTAKE

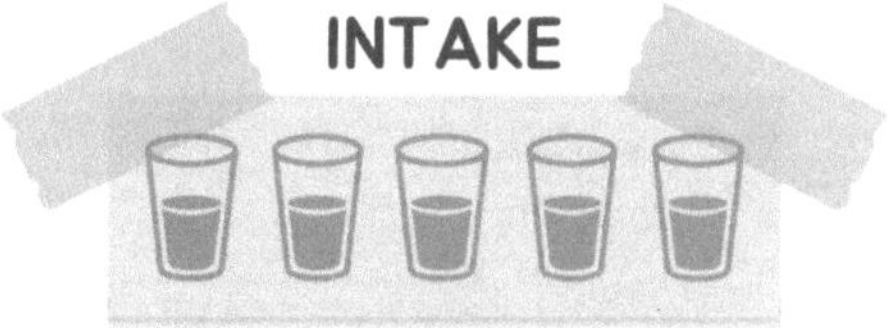

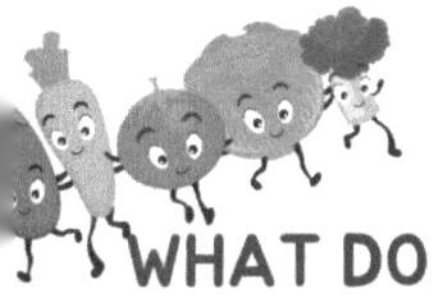

WHAT DOES YOUR MEAL LOOK LIKE TODAY

Breakfast:

Lunch:

Dinner:

Snack:

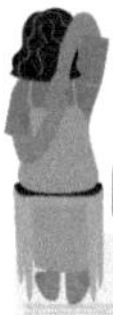

HOW WERE YOUR MOVEMENTS TODAY?

LETS GO THROUGH THE CHECKLIST DAY 10

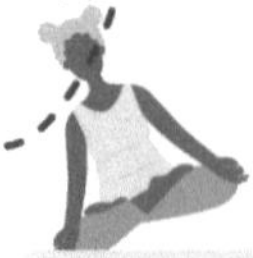

DID YOU MEDITATE?

HOW LONG?

HOW DO YOU FEEL?

DID YOU MAKE SURE TO BREATHE?

DON'T FORGET YOUR MANTRAS.

MEDS AND HERBS INTAKE

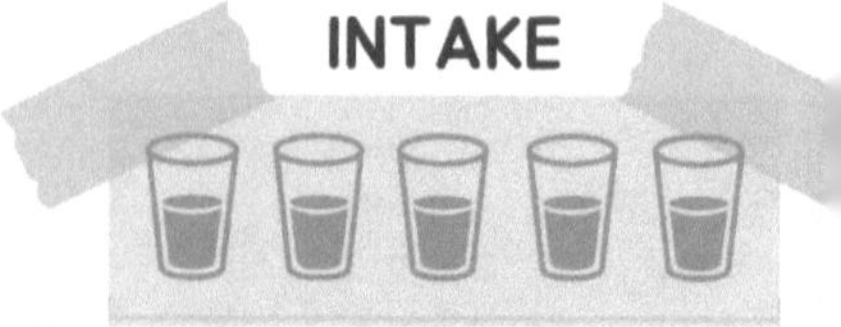

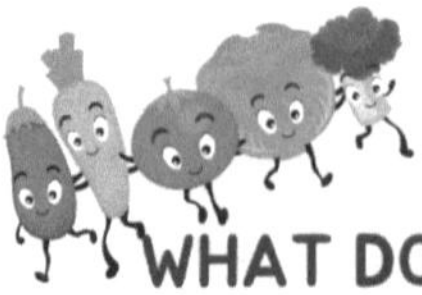

WHAT DOES YOUR MEAL LOOK LIKE TODAY

Breakfast:

Lunch:

Dinner:

Snack:

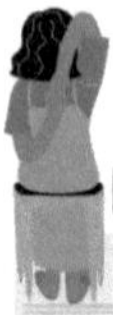

HOW WERE YOUR MOVEMENTS TODAY?

LETS GO THROUGH THE CHECKLIST DAY 11

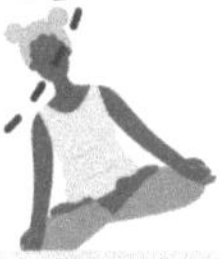

DID YOU MEDITATE?

HOW LONG?

HOW DO YOU FEEL?

DID YOU MAKE SURE TO BREATHE?

DON'T FORGET YOUR MANTRAS.

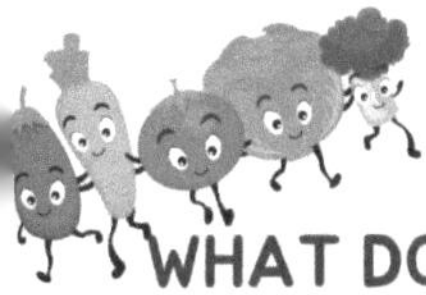

WHAT DOES YOUR MEAL LOOK LIKE TODAY

Breakfast:

Lunch:

Dinner:

Snack:

MEDS AND HERBS INTAKE

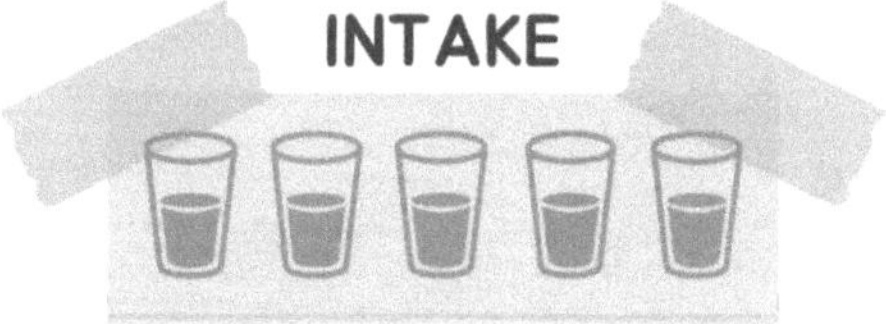

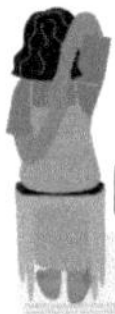

HOW WERE YOUR MOVEMENTS TODAY?

LETS GO THROUGH THE CHECKLIST DAY 12

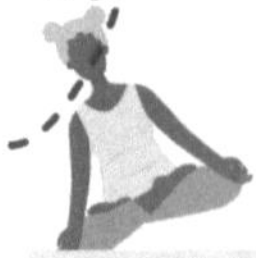

DID YOU MEDITATE?

HOW LONG?

HOW DO YOU FEEL?

DID YOU MAKE SURE TO BREATHE?

DON'T FORGET YOUR MANTRAS.

MEDS AND HERBS INTAKE

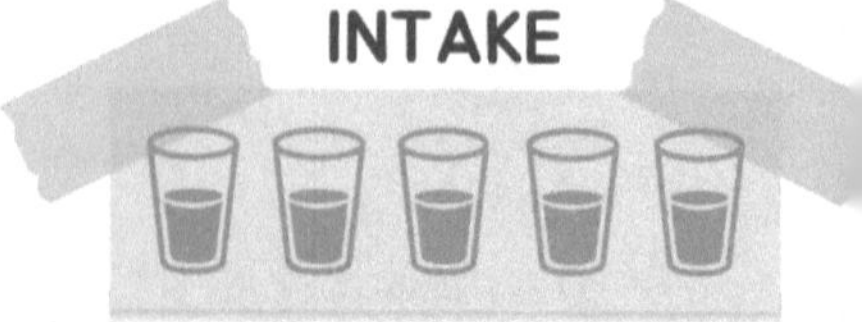

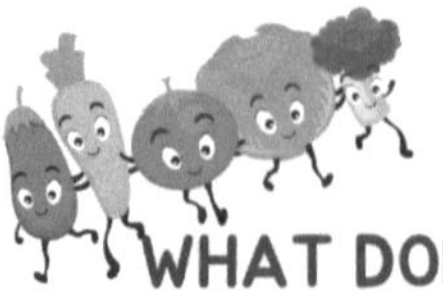

WHAT DOES YOUR MEAL LOOK LIKE TODAY

Breakfast:

Lunch:

Dinner:

Snack:

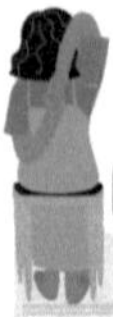

HOW WERE YOUR MOVEMENTS TODAY?

LETS GO THROUGH THE CHECKLIST DAY 13

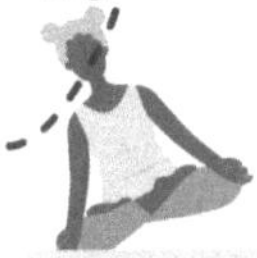

DID YOU MEDITATE?

HOW LONG?

HOW DO YOU FEEL?

DID YOU MAKE SURE TO BREATHE?

DON'T FORGET YOUR MANTRAS.

MEDS AND HERBS INTAKE

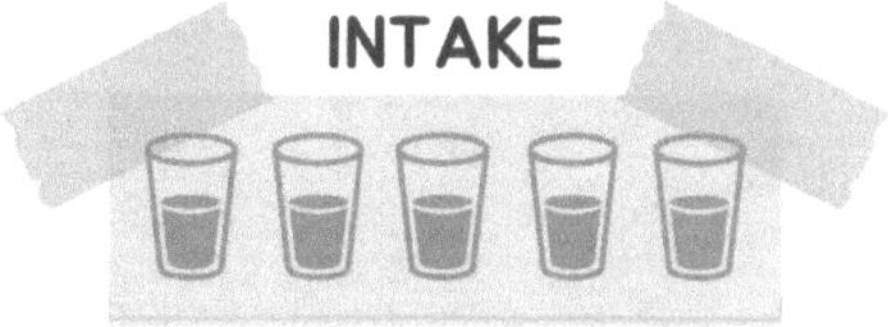

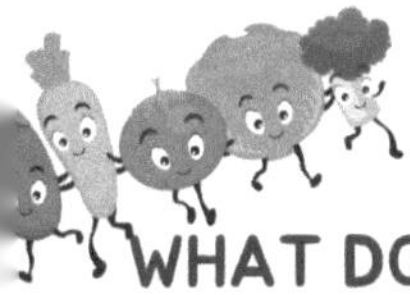

WHAT DOES YOUR MEAL LOOK LIKE TODAY

Breakfast:

Lunch:

Dinner:

Snack:

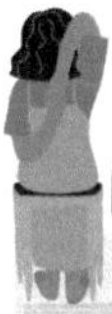

HOW WERE YOUR MOVEMENTS TODAY?

LETS GO THROUGH THE CHECKLIST DAY 14

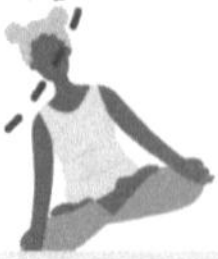

DID YOU MEDITATE?

HOW LONG?

HOW DO YOU FEEL?

DID YOU MAKE SURE TO BREATHE?

DON'T FORGET YOUR MANTRAS.

MEDS AND HERBS INTAKE

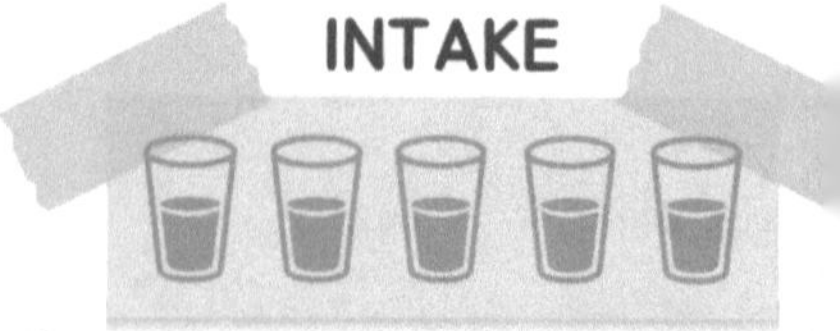

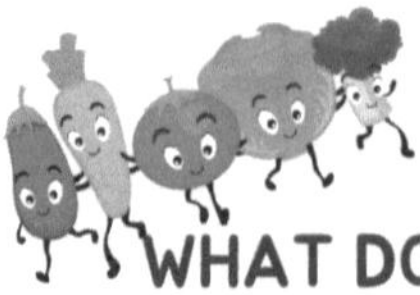

WHAT DOES YOUR MEAL LOOK LIKE TODAY

Breakfast:

Lunch:

Dinner:

Snack:

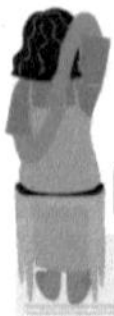

HOW WERE YOUR MOVEMENTS TODAY?

ANOTHER WEEK

WHEEW!

I KNOW ITS STILL

A CHALLENGE BUT

LETS MOVE AND

STRETCH

AT YOUR PACE

OF COURSE BUT

EVERYDAY!.

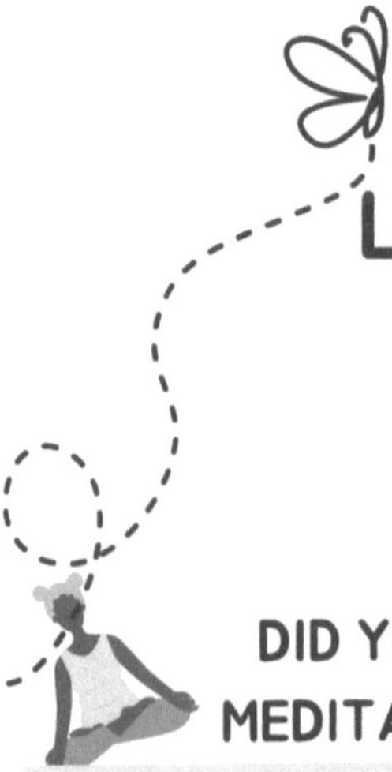

LETS GO THROUGH THE CHECKLIST DAY 15

DID YOU MEDITATE?

HOW LONG?

HOW DO YOU FEEL?

DID YOU MAKE SURE TO BREATHE?

DON'T FORGET YOUR MANTRAS.

MEDS AND HERBS INTAKE

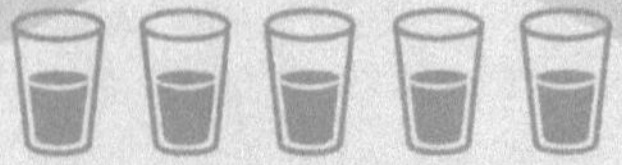

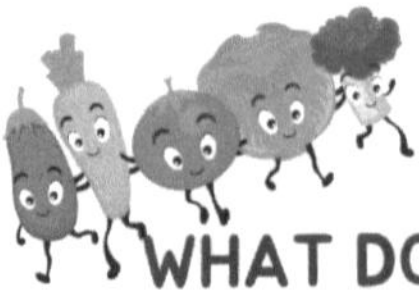

WHAT DOES YOUR MEAL LOOK LIKE TODAY

Breakfast:

Lunch:

Dinner:

Snack:

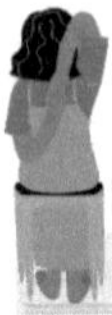

HOW WERE YOUR MOVEMENTS TODAY?

LETS GO THROUGH THE CHECKLIST DAY 16

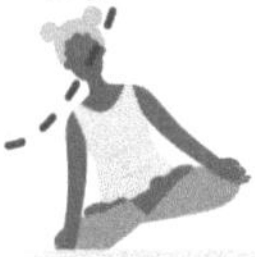

DID YOU MEDITATE?

HOW LONG?

HOW DO YOU FEEL?

DID YOU MAKE SURE TO BREATHE?

DON'T FORGET YOUR MANTRAS.

MEDS AND HERBS INTAKE

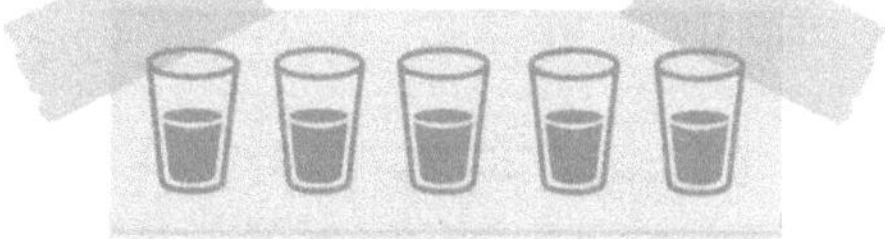

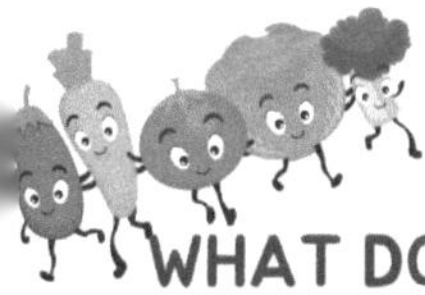

WHAT DOES YOUR MEAL LOOK LIKE TODAY

Breakfast:

Lunch:

Dinner:

Snack:

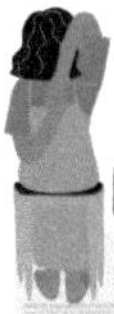

HOW WERE YOUR MOVEMENTS TODAY?

LETS GO THROUGH THE CHECKLIST
DAY 17

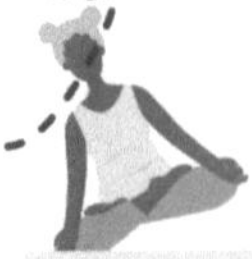

DID YOU MEDITATE?

HOW LONG?

HOW DO YOU FEEL?

DID YOU MAKE SURE TO BREATHE?

DON'T FORGET YOUR MANTRAS.

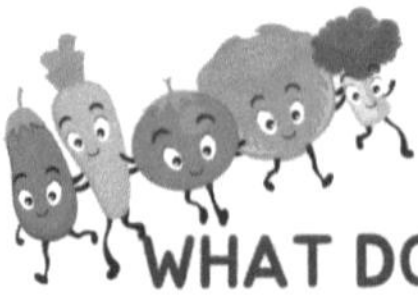

WHAT DOES YOUR MEAL LOOK LIKE TODAY

Breakfast:

Lunch:

Dinner:

Snack:

MEDS AND HERBS INTAKE

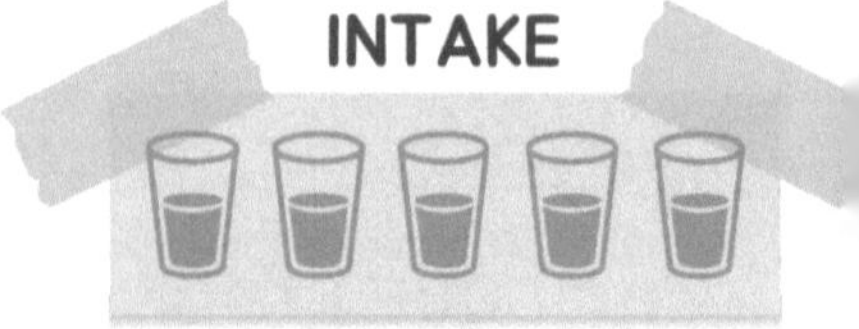

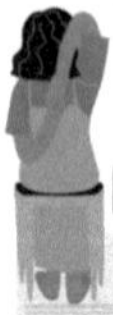

HOW WERE YOUR MOVEMENTS TODAY?

LETS GO THROUGH THE CHECKLIST DAY 18

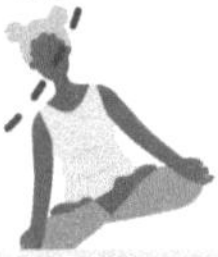

DID YOU MEDITATE?

HOW LONG?

HOW DO YOU FEEL?

DID YOU MAKE SURE TO BREATHE?

DON'T FORGET YOUR MANTRAS.

MEDS AND HERBS INTAKE

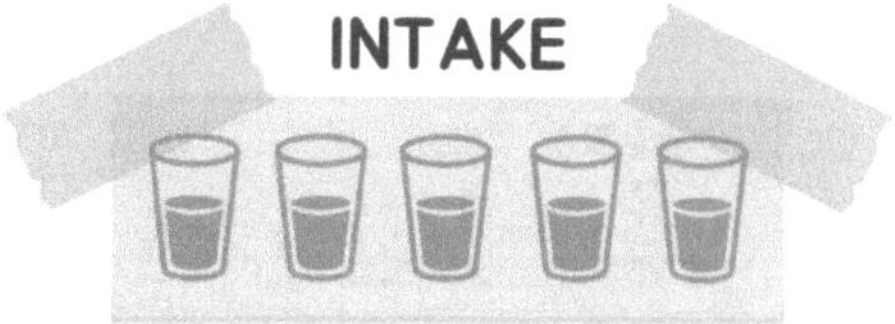

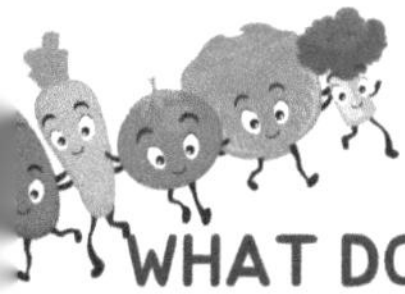

WHAT DOES YOUR MEAL LOOK LIKE TODAY

Breakfast:

Lunch:

Dinner:

Snack:

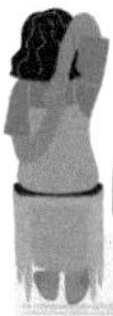

HOW WERE YOUR MOVEMENTS TODAY?

LETS GO THROUGH THE CHECKLIST DAY 19

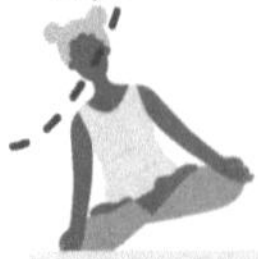

DID YOU MEDITATE?

HOW LONG?

HOW DO YOU FEEL?

DID YOU MAKE SURE TO BREATHE?

DON'T FORGET YOUR MANTRAS.

MEDS AND HERBS INTAKE

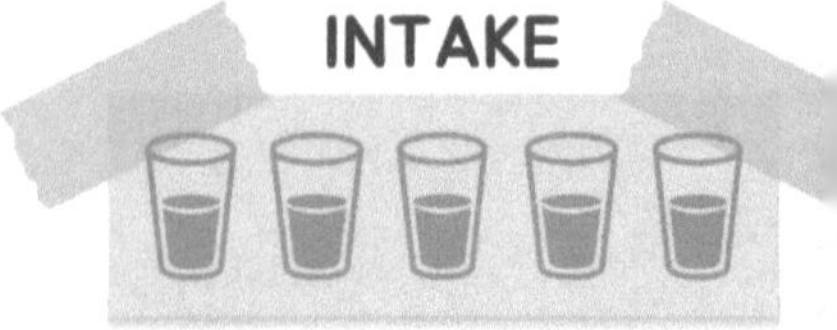

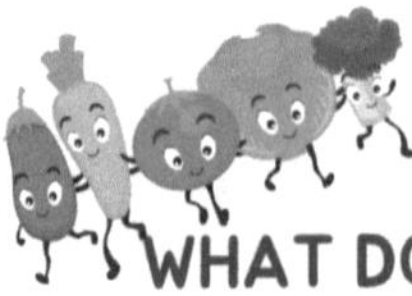

WHAT DOES YOUR MEAL LOOK LIKE TODAY

Breakfast:

Lunch:

Dinner:

Snack:

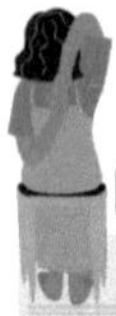

HOW WERE YOUR MOVEMENTS TODAY?

LETS GO THROUGH THE CHECKLIST DAY 20

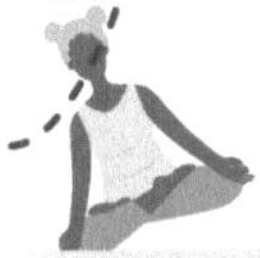

DID YOU MEDITATE?

HOW LONG?

HOW DO YOU FEEL?

DID YOU MAKE SURE TO BREATHE?

DON'T FORGET YOUR MANTRAS.

MEDS AND HERBS INTAKE

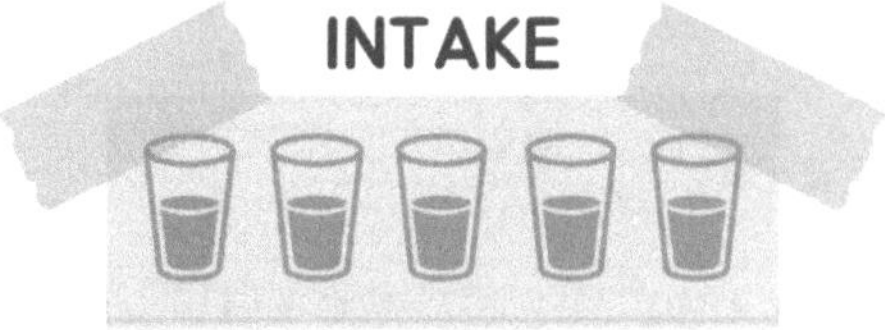

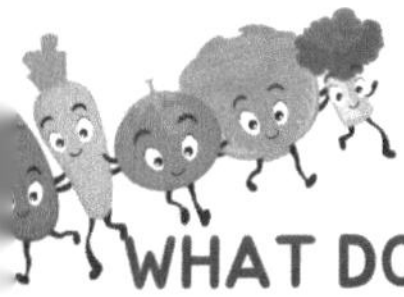

WHAT DOES YOUR MEAL LOOK LIKE TODAY

Breakfast:

Lunch:

Dinner:

Snack:

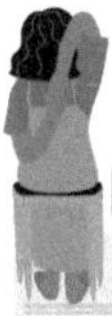

HOW WERE YOUR MOVEMENTS TODAY?

LETS GO THROUGH THE CHECKLIST DAY 21

DID YOU MEDITATE?

HOW LONG?

HOW DO YOU FEEL?

DID YOU MAKE SURE TO BREATHE?

DON'T FORGET YOUR MANTRAS.

MEDS AND HERBS INTAKE

WHAT DOES YOUR MEAL LOOK LIKE TODAY

Breakfast:

Lunch:

Dinner:

Snack:

HOW WERE YOUR MOVEMENTS TODAY?

HAVE YOU BEEN EATING
RIGHT?
GETTING THOSE
VEGGIES
AND FRUITS IN?
LOTS OF WATER,
REHYDRATE YOURSELF,
SURGERY TAKES A LOT
OUT OF YOU! YOU HAVE
TO PUT IT BACK!

LETS GO THROUGH THE CHECKLIST DAY 22

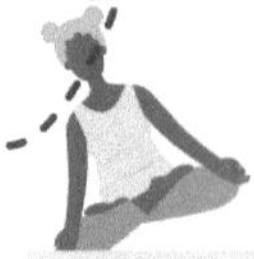

DID YOU MEDITATE?

HOW LONG?

HOW DO YOU FEEL?

DID YOU MAKE SURE TO BREATHE?

DON'T FORGET YOUR MANTRAS.

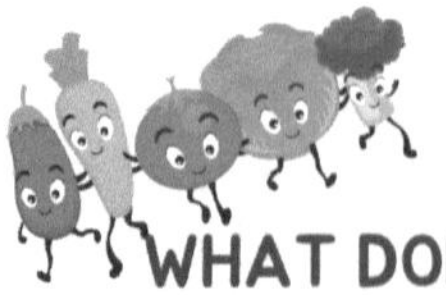

WHAT DOES YOUR MEAL LOOK LIKE TODAY

Breakfast:

Lunch:

Dinner:

Snack:

MEDS AND HERBS INTAKE

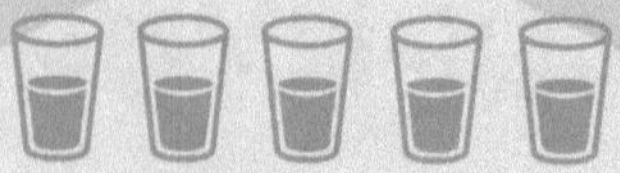

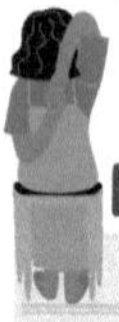

HOW WERE YOUR MOVEMENTS TODAY?

LETS GO THROUGH THE CHECKLIST DAY 23

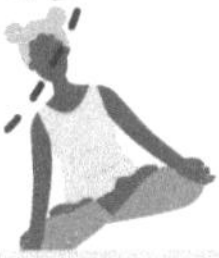

DID YOU MEDITATE?

HOW LONG?

HOW DO YOU FEEL?

DID YOU MAKE SURE TO BREATHE?

DON'T FORGET YOUR MANTRAS.

MEDS AND HERBS INTAKE

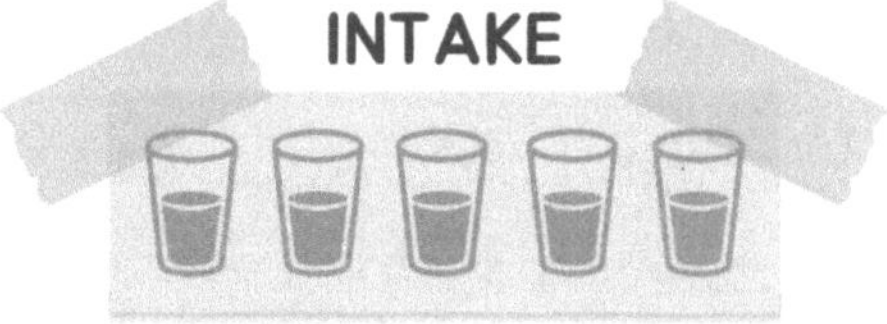

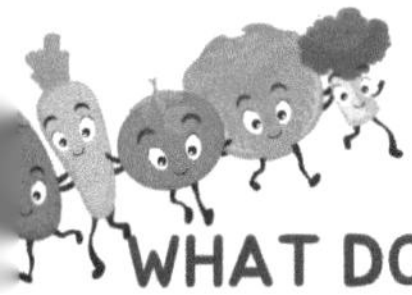

WHAT DOES YOUR MEAL LOOK LIKE TODAY

Breakfast:

Lunch:

Dinner:

Snack:

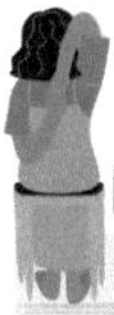

HOW WERE YOUR MOVEMENTS TODAY?

LETS GO THROUGH THE CHECKLIST DAY 24

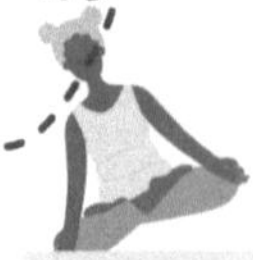

DID YOU MEDITATE?

HOW LONG?

HOW DO YOU FEEL?

DID YOU MAKE SURE TO BREATHE?

DON'T FORGET YOUR MANTRAS.

MEDS AND HERBS INTAKE

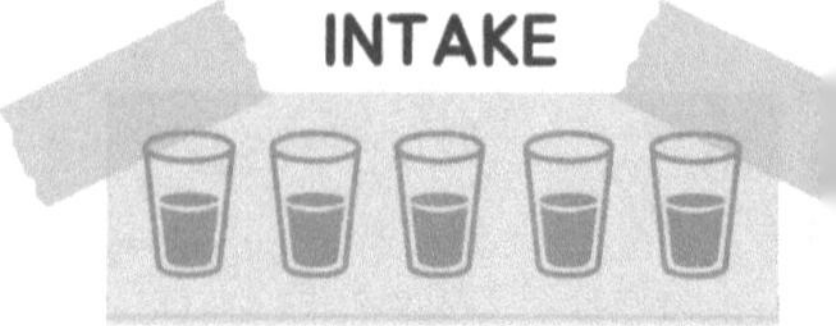

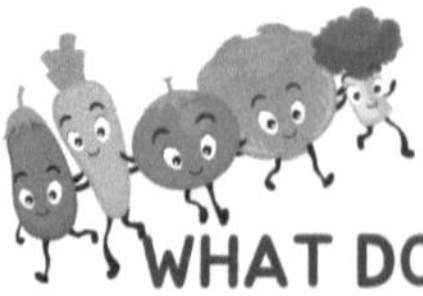

WHAT DOES YOUR MEAL LOOK LIKE TODAY

Breakfast:

Lunch:

Dinner:

Snack:

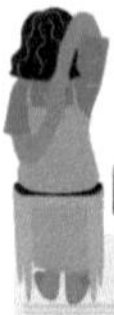

HOW WERE YOUR MOVEMENTS TODAY?

LETS GO THROUGH THE CHECKLIST DAY 25

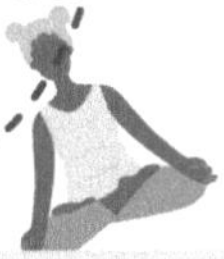

DID YOU MEDITATE?

HOW LONG?

HOW DO YOU FEEL?

DID YOU MAKE SURE TO BREATHE?

DON'T FORGET YOUR MANTRAS.

MEDS AND HERBS INTAKE

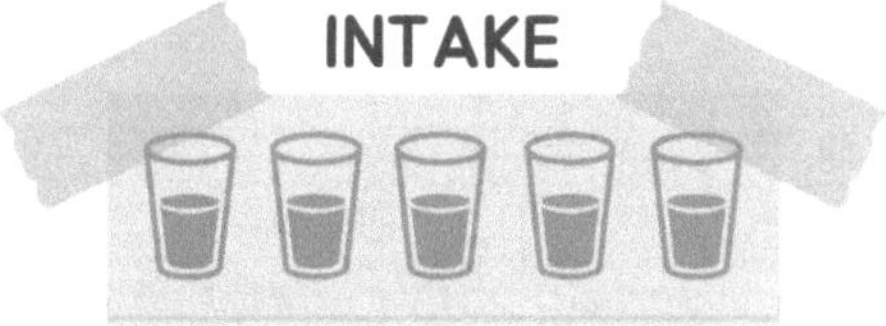

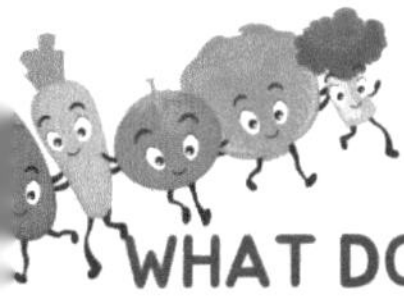

WHAT DOES YOUR MEAL LOOK LIKE TODAY

Breakfast:

Lunch:

Dinner:

Snack:

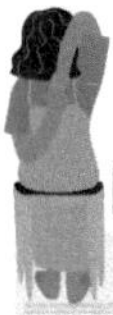

HOW WERE YOUR MOVEMENTS TODAY?

LETS GO THROUGH THE CHECKLIST DAY 26

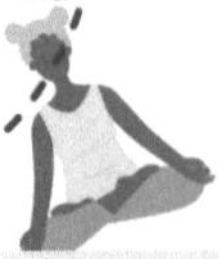

DID YOU MEDITATE?

HOW LONG?

HOW DO YOU FEEL?

DID YOU MAKE SURE TO BREATHE?

DON'T FORGET YOUR MANTRAS.

MEDS AND HERBS INTAKE

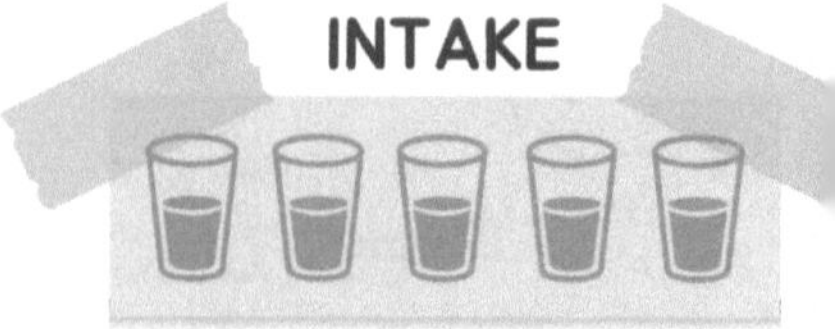

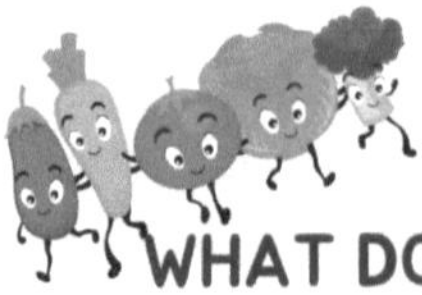

WHAT DOES YOUR MEAL LOOK LIKE TODAY

Breakfast:

Lunch:

Dinner:

Snack:

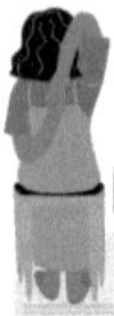

HOW WERE YOUR MOVEMENTS TODAY?

LETS GO THROUGH THE CHECKLIST

DAY 27

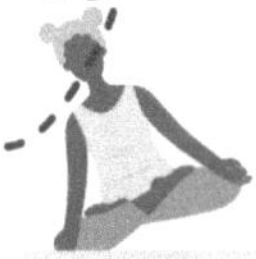

DID YOU MEDITATE?

HOW LONG?

HOW DO YOU FEEL?

DID YOU MAKE SURE TO BREATHE?

DON'T FORGET YOUR MANTRAS.

MEDS AND HERBS INTAKE

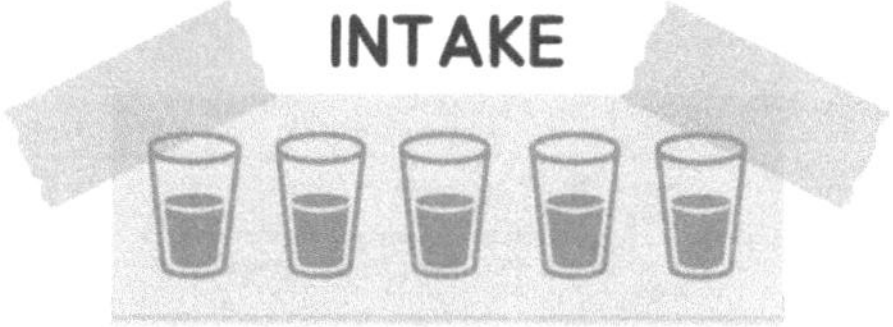

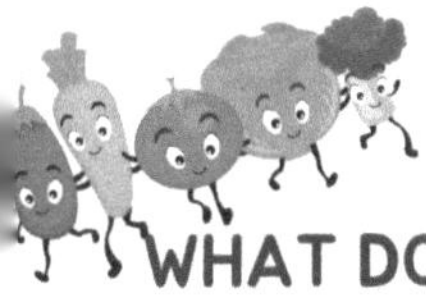

WHAT DOES YOUR MEAL LOOK LIKE TODAY

Breakfast:

Lunch:

Dinner:

Snack:

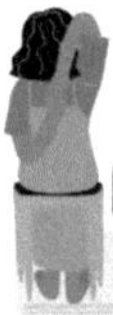

HOW WERE YOUR MOVEMENTS TODAY?

LETS GO THROUGH THE CHECKLIST DAY 28

DID YOU MEDITATE?

HOW LONG?

HOW DO YOU FEEL?

DID YOU MAKE SURE TO BREATHE?

DON'T FORGET YOUR MANTRAS.

MEDS AND HERBS INTAKE

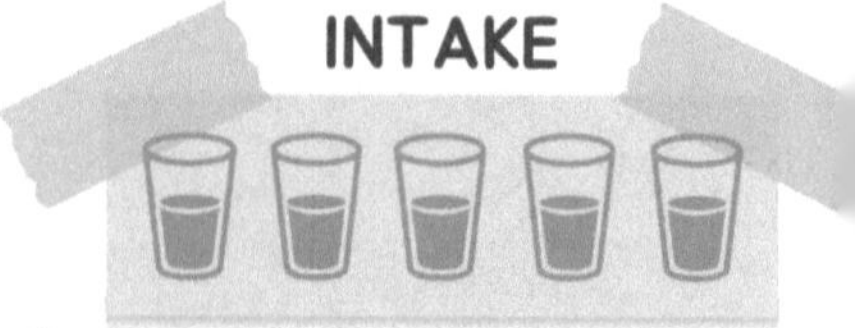

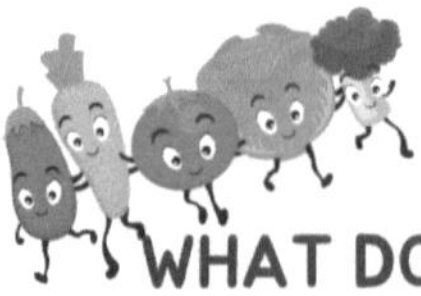

WHAT DOES YOUR MEAL LOOK LIKE TODAY

Breakfast:

Lunch:

Dinner:

Snack:

HOW WERE YOUR MOVEMENTS TODAY?

DON'T FORGET TO
MOTIVATE
YOURSELF!
LOOK IN THAT
MIRROR AND
EMBRACE IT.
YOU ARE ABLE!
YOU ARE BEAUTIFUL!
YOU ARE A BETTER
YOU!

LETS GO THROUGH THE CHECKLIST DAY 29

DID YOU MEDITATE?

HOW LONG?

HOW DO YOU FEEL?

DID YOU MAKE SURE TO BREATHE?

DON'T FORGET YOUR MANTRAS.

MEDS AND HERBS INTAKE

WHAT DOES YOUR MEAL LOOK LIKE TODAY

Breakfast:

Lunch:

Dinner:

Snack:

HOW WERE YOUR MOVEMENTS TODAY?

LETS GO THROUGH THE CHECKLIST DAY 30

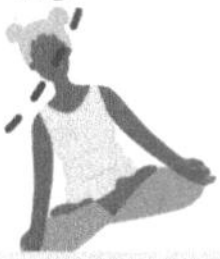

DID YOU MEDITATE?

HOW LONG?

HOW DO YOU FEEL?

DID YOU MAKE SURE TO BREATHE?

DON'T FORGET YOUR MANTRAS.

MEDS AND HERBS INTAKE

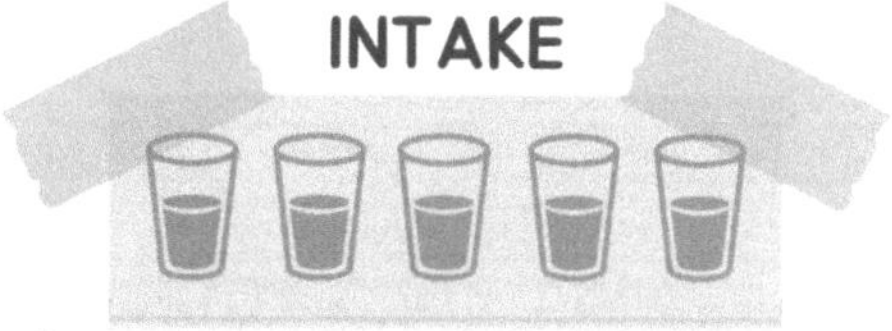

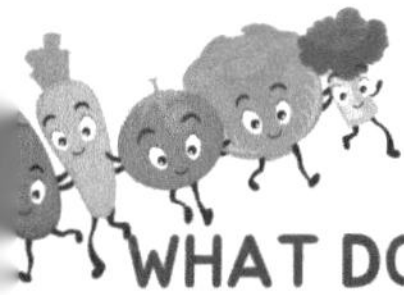

WHAT DOES YOUR MEAL LOOK LIKE TODAY

Breakfast:

Lunch:

Dinner:

Snack:

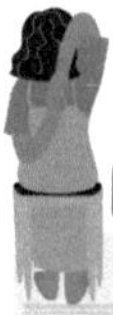

HOW WERE YOUR MOVEMENTS TODAY?

LETS GO THROUGH THE CHECKLIST DAY 31

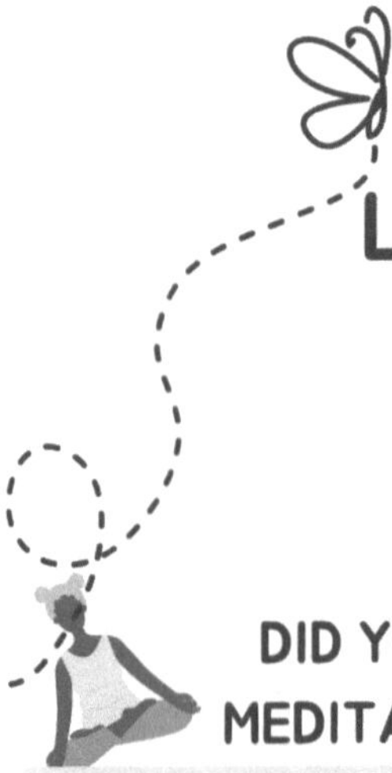

DID YOU MEDITATE?

HOW LONG?

HOW DO YOU FEEL?

DID YOU MAKE SURE TO BREATHE?

DON'T FORGET YOUR MANTRAS.

MEDS AND HERBS INTAKE

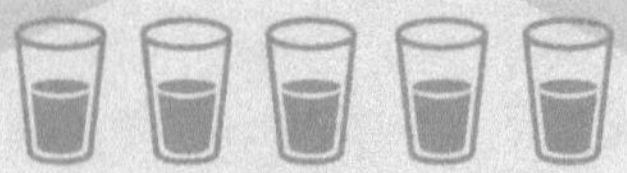

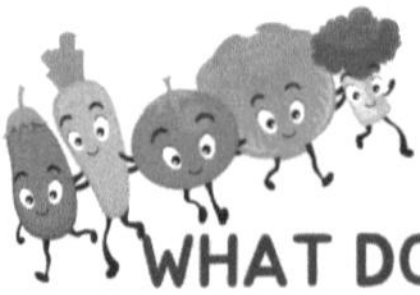

WHAT DOES YOUR MEAL LOOK LIKE TODAY

Breakfast:

Lunch:

Dinner:

Snack:

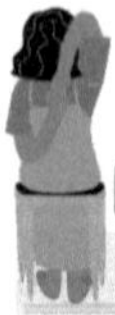

HOW WERE YOUR MOVEMENTS TODAY?

LETS GO THROUGH THE CHECKLIST DAY 32

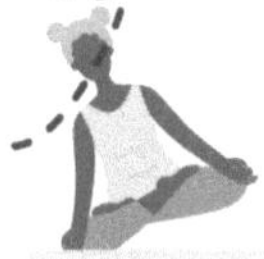

DID YOU MEDITATE?

HOW LONG?

HOW DO YOU FEEL?

DID YOU MAKE SURE TO BREATHE?

DON'T FORGET YOUR MANTRAS.

MEDS AND HERBS INTAKE

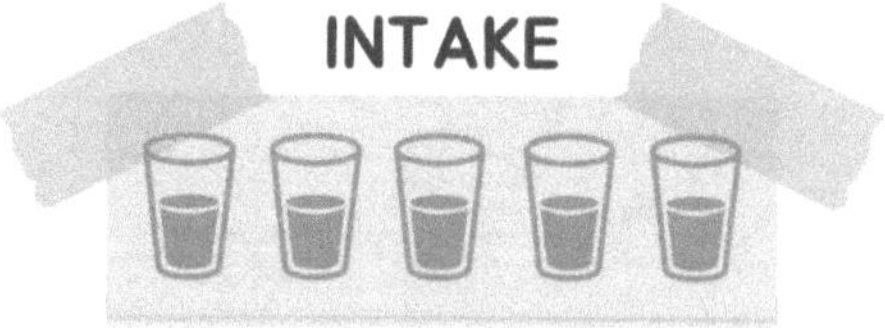

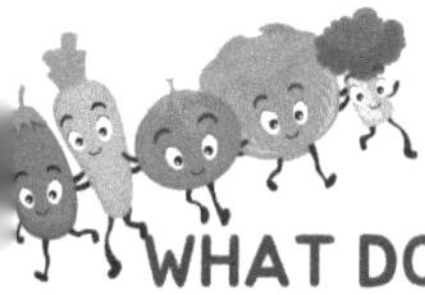

WHAT DOES YOUR MEAL LOOK LIKE TODAY

Breakfast:

Lunch:

Dinner:

Snack:

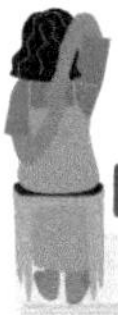

HOW WERE YOUR MOVEMENTS TODAY?

LETS GO THROUGH THE CHECKLIST DAY 33

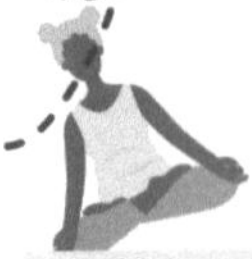

DID YOU MEDITATE?

HOW LONG?

HOW DO YOU FEEL?

DID YOU MAKE SURE TO BREATHE?

DON'T FORGET YOUR MANTRAS.

MEDS AND HERBS INTAKE

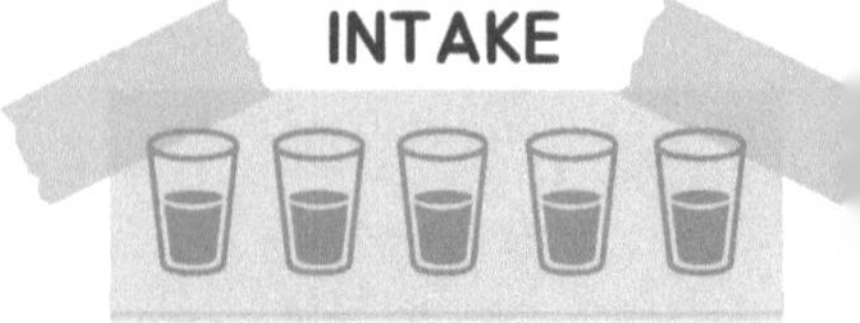

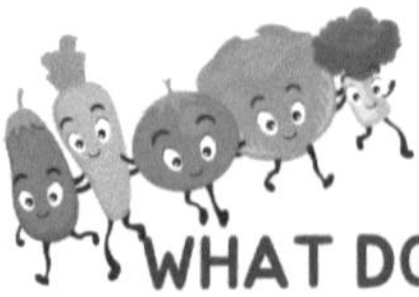

WHAT DOES YOUR MEAL LOOK LIKE TODAY

Breakfast:

Lunch:

Dinner:

Snack:

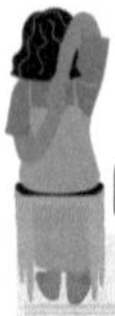

HOW WERE YOUR MOVEMENTS TODAY?

LETS GO THROUGH THE CHECKLIST DAY 34

DID YOU MEDITATE?

HOW LONG?

HOW DO YOU FEEL?

DID YOU MAKE SURE TO BREATHE?

DON'T FORGET YOUR MANTRAS.

MEDS AND HERBS INTAKE

WHAT DOES YOUR MEAL LOOK LIKE TODAY

Breakfast:

Lunch:

Dinner:

Snack:

HOW WERE YOUR MOVEMENTS TODAY?

LETS GO THROUGH THE CHECKLIST DAY 35

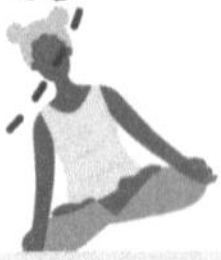

DID YOU MEDITATE?

HOW LONG?

HOW DO YOU FEEL?

DID YOU MAKE SURE TO BREATHE?

DON'T FORGET YOUR MANTRAS.

MEDS AND HERBS INTAKE

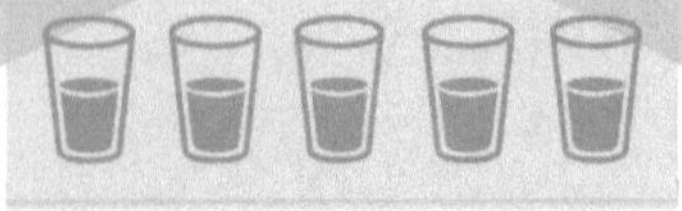

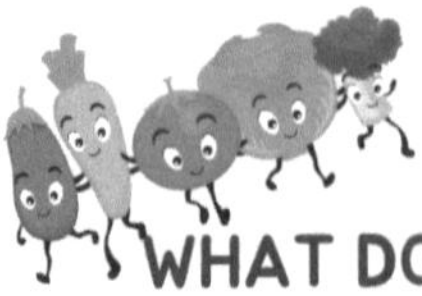

WHAT DOES YOUR MEAL LOOK LIKE TODAY

Breakfast:

Lunch:

Dinner:

Snack:

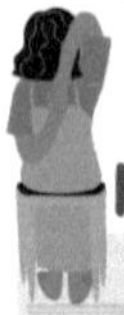

HOW WERE YOUR MOVEMENTS TODAY?

ARE YOU ABLE TO
SEE THE SUN FROM
YOUR HOME?
MAKE SURE TO LET
IT HIT YOUR SKIN
AND BREATHE IN,
BREATHE OUT AND
THANK YOURSELF
FOR LOVING YOU!
THANK THE SUN FOR
GIVING YOU ENERGY!

LETS GO THROUGH THE CHECKLIST DAY 36

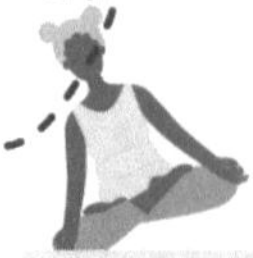

DID YOU MEDITATE?

HOW LONG?

HOW DO YOU FEEL?

DID YOU MAKE SURE TO BREATHE?

DON'T FORGET YOUR MANTRAS.

MEDS AND HERBS INTAKE

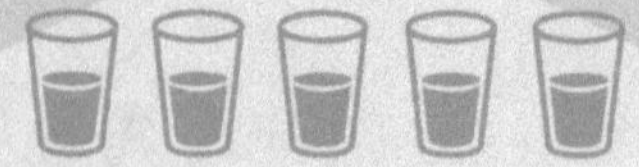

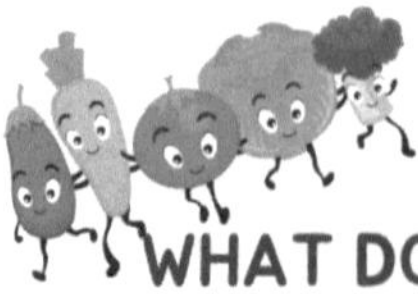

WHAT DOES YOUR MEAL LOOK LIKE TODAY

Breakfast:

Lunch:

Dinner:

Snack:

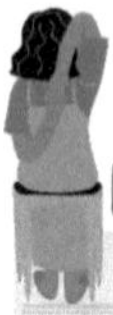

HOW WERE YOUR MOVEMENTS TODAY?

LETS GO THROUGH THE CHECKLIST DAY 37

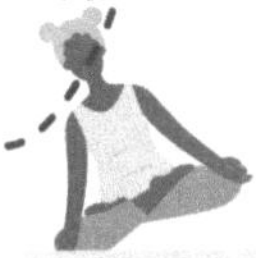

DID YOU MEDITATE?

HOW LONG?

HOW DO YOU FEEL?

DID YOU MAKE SURE TO BREATHE?

DON'T FORGET YOUR MANTRAS.

MEDS AND HERBS INTAKE

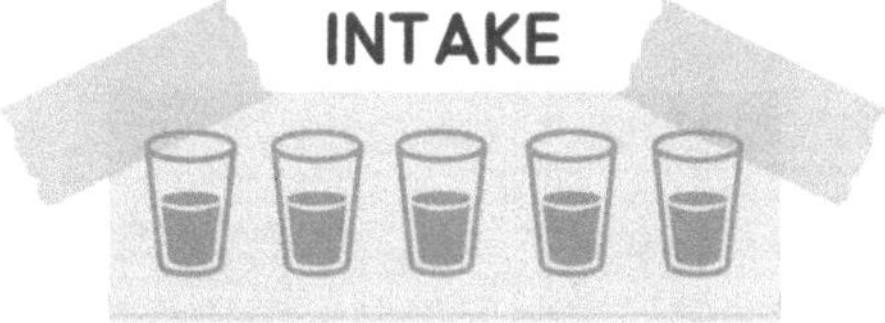

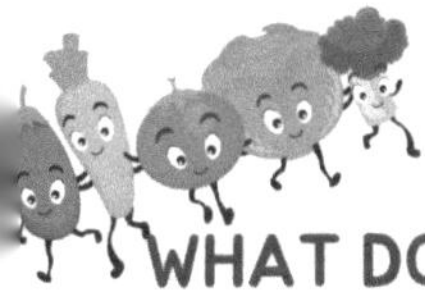

WHAT DOES YOUR MEAL LOOK LIKE TODAY

Breakfast:

Lunch:

Dinner:

Snack:

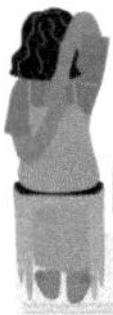

HOW WERE YOUR MOVEMENTS TODAY?

LETS GO THROUGH THE CHECKLIST DAY 38

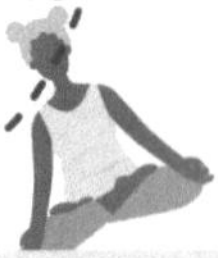

DID YOU MEDITATE?

HOW LONG?

HOW DO YOU FEEL?

DID YOU MAKE SURE TO BREATHE?

DON'T FORGET YOUR MANTRAS.

MEDS AND HERBS INTAKE

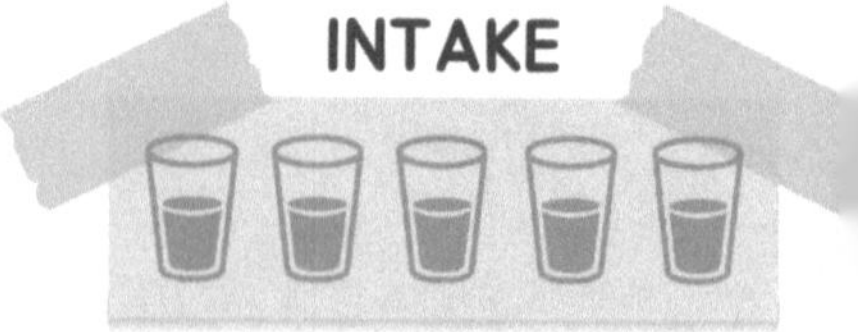

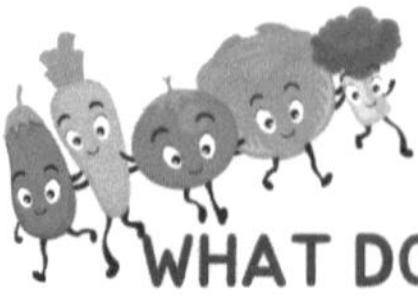

WHAT DOES YOUR MEAL LOOK LIKE TODAY

Breakfast:

Lunch:

Dinner:

Snack:

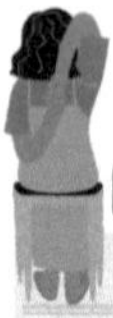

HOW WERE YOUR MOVEMENTS TODAY?

LETS GO THROUGH THE CHECKLIST DAY 39

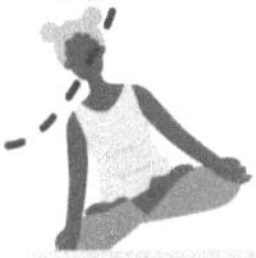

DID YOU MEDITATE?

HOW LONG?

HOW DO YOU FEEL?

DID YOU MAKE SURE TO BREATHE?

DON'T FORGET YOUR MANTRAS.

MEDS AND HERBS INTAKE

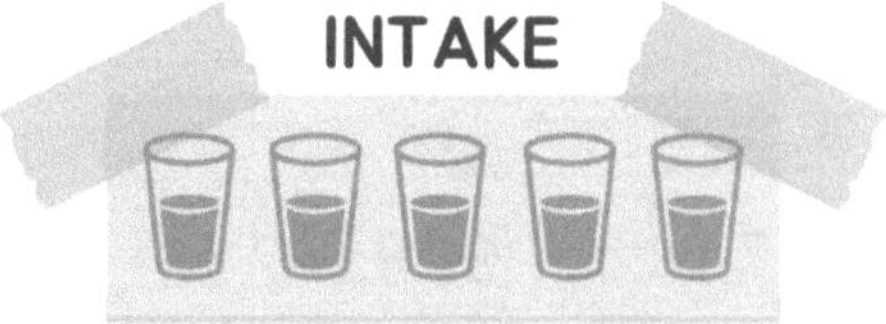

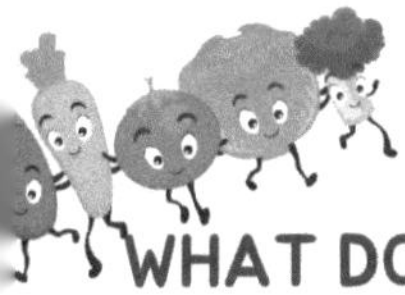

WHAT DOES YOUR MEAL LOOK LIKE TODAY

Breakfast:

Lunch:

Dinner:

Snack:

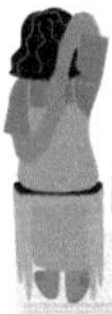

HOW WERE YOUR MOVEMENTS TODAY?

LETS GO THROUGH THE CHECKLIST DAY 40

DID YOU MEDITATE?

HOW LONG?

HOW DO YOU FEEL?

DID YOU MAKE SURE TO BREATHE?

DON'T FORGET YOUR MANTRAS.

MEDS AND HERBS INTAKE

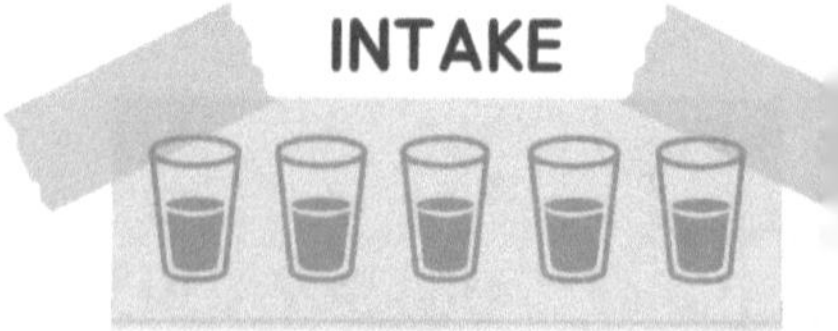

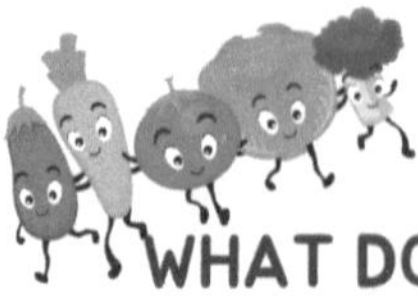

WHAT DOES YOUR MEAL LOOK LIKE TODAY

Breakfast:

Lunch:

Dinner:

Snack:

HOW WERE YOUR MOVEMENTS TODAY?

LETS GO THROUGH THE CHECKLIST DAY 41

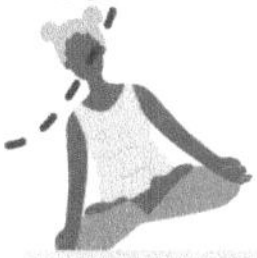

DID YOU MEDITATE?

HOW LONG?

HOW DO YOU FEEL?

DID YOU MAKE SURE TO BREATHE?

DON'T FORGET YOUR MANTRAS.

MEDS AND HERBS INTAKE

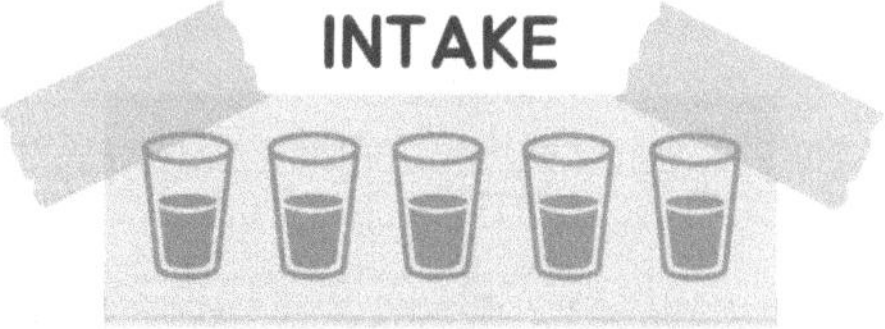

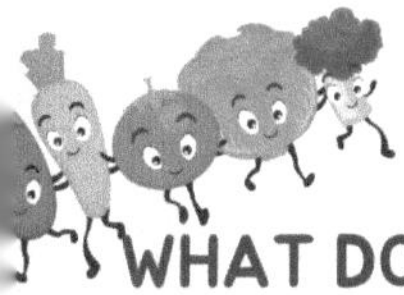

WHAT DOES YOUR MEAL LOOK LIKE TODAY

Breakfast:

Lunch:

Dinner:

Snack:

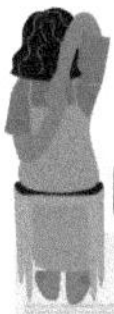

HOW WERE YOUR MOVEMENTS TODAY?

LETS GO THROUGH THE CHECKLIST DAY 42

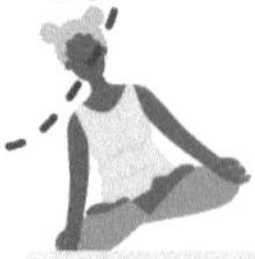

DID YOU MEDITATE?

HOW LONG?

HOW DO YOU FEEL?

DID YOU MAKE SURE TO BREATHE?

DON'T FORGET YOUR MANTRAS.

MEDS AND HERBS INTAKE

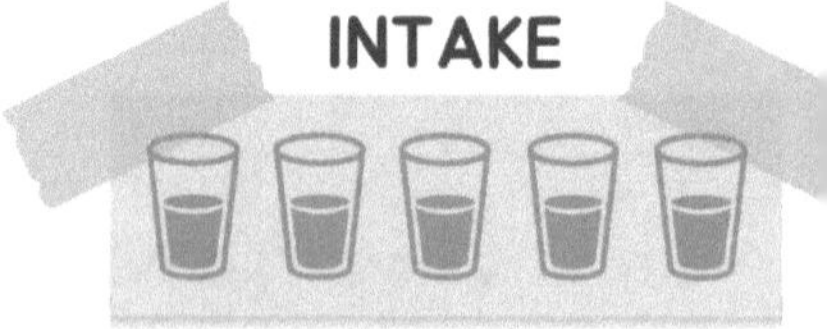

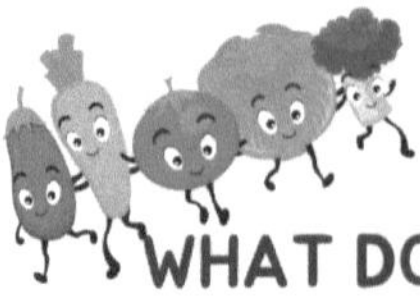

WHAT DOES YOUR MEAL LOOK LIKE TODAY

Breakfast:

Lunch:

Dinner:

Snack:

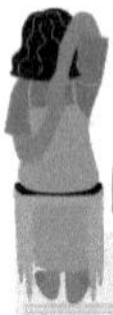

HOW WERE YOUR MOVEMENTS TODAY?

THIS IS YOUR
SECOND MONTH.
DON'T RUSH TO GO
OUTSIDE IF YOU DO
NOT HAVE TO!
STAY HOME AND SIT
STILL!
SITTING STILL
PROVIDES A PEACE
THAT IS TRULY
INDESCRIBABLE!

LETS GO THROUGH THE CHECKLIST DAY 43

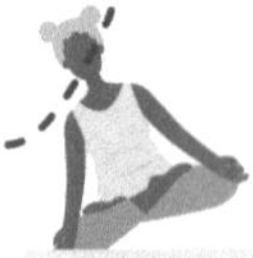

DID YOU MEDITATE?

HOW LONG?

HOW DO YOU FEEL?

DID YOU MAKE SURE TO BREATHE?

DON'T FORGET YOUR MANTRAS.

MEDS AND HERBS INTAKE

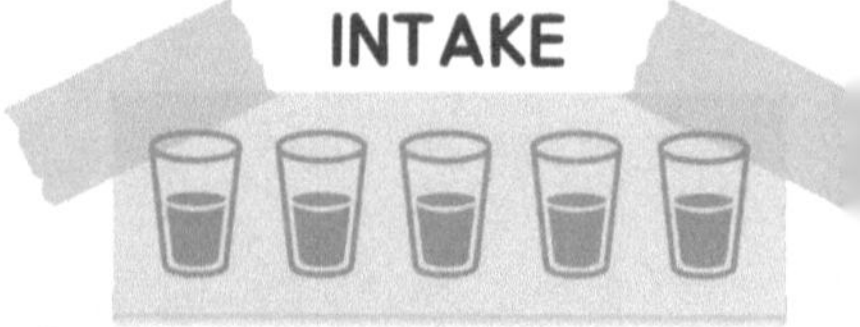

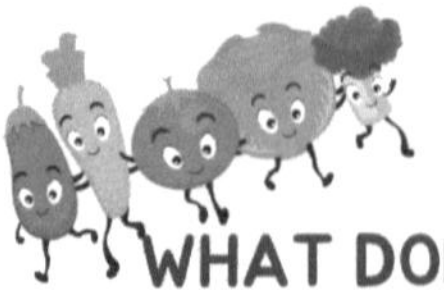

WHAT DOES YOUR MEAL LOOK LIKE TODAY

Breakfast:

Lunch:

Dinner:

Snack:

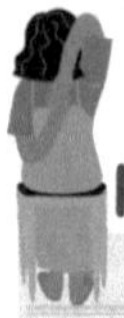

HOW WERE YOUR MOVEMENTS TODAY?

LETS GO THROUGH THE CHECKLIST DAY 44

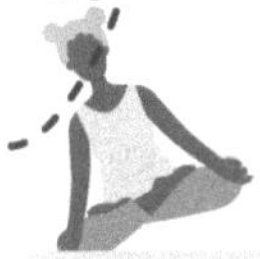

DID YOU MEDITATE?

HOW LONG?

HOW DO YOU FEEL?

DID YOU MAKE SURE TO BREATHE?

DON'T FORGET YOUR MANTRAS.

MEDS AND HERBS INTAKE

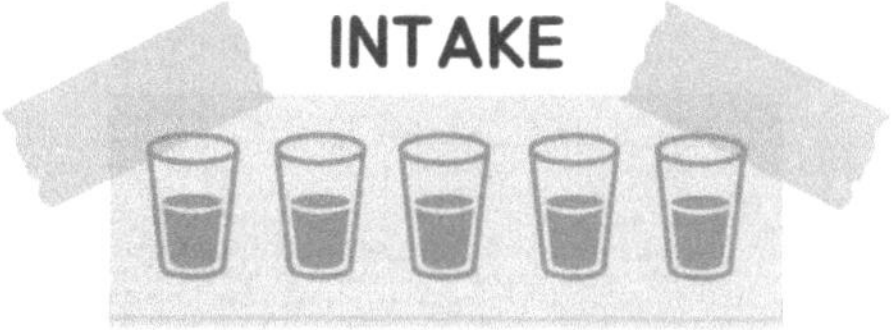

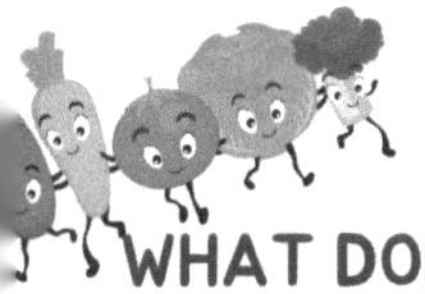

WHAT DOES YOUR MEAL LOOK LIKE TODAY

Breakfast:

Lunch:

Dinner:

Snack:

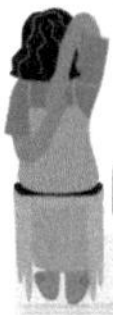

HOW WERE YOUR MOVEMENTS TODAY?

LETS GO THROUGH THE CHECKLIST DAY 45

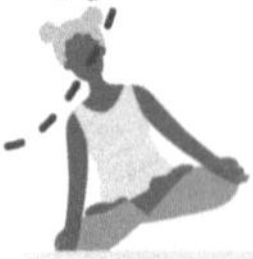

DID YOU MEDITATE?

HOW LONG?

HOW DO YOU FEEL?

DID YOU MAKE SURE TO BREATHE?

DON'T FORGET YOUR MANTRAS.

MEDS AND HERBS INTAKE

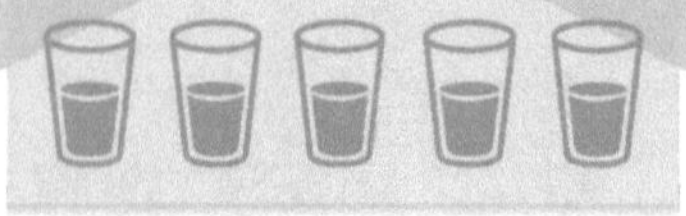

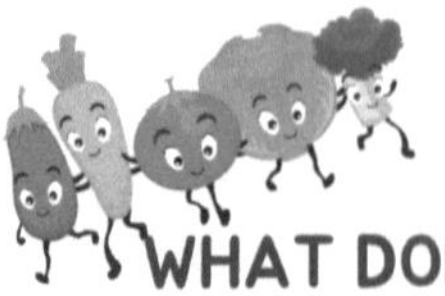

WHAT DOES YOUR MEAL LOOK LIKE TODAY

Breakfast:

Lunch:

Dinner:

Snack:

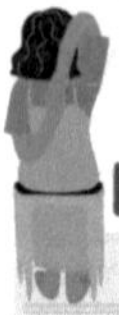

HOW WERE YOUR MOVEMENTS TODAY?

LETS GO THROUGH THE CHECKLIST DAY 46

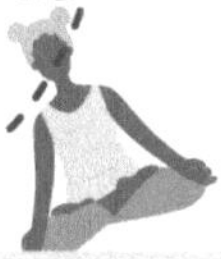

DID YOU MEDITATE?

HOW LONG?

HOW DO YOU FEEL?

DID YOU MAKE SURE TO BREATHE?

DON'T FORGET YOUR MANTRAS.

MEDS AND HERBS INTAKE

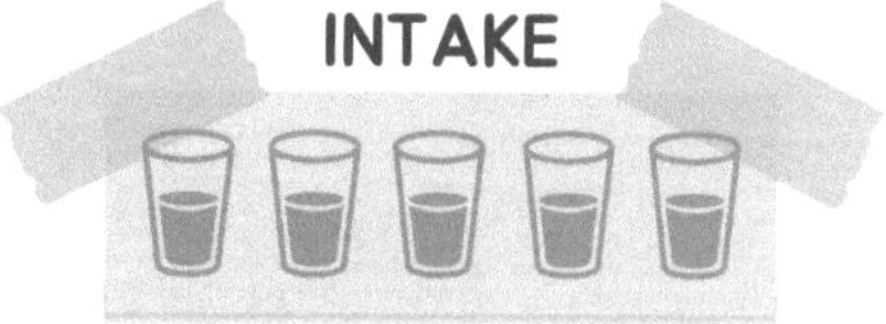

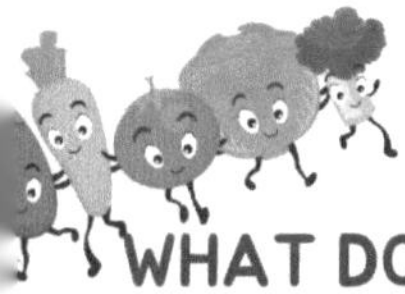

WHAT DOES YOUR MEAL LOOK LIKE TODAY

Breakfast:

Lunch:

Dinner:

Snack:

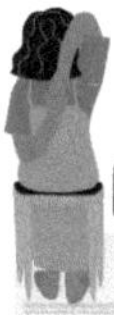

HOW WERE YOUR MOVEMENTS TODAY?

LETS GO THROUGH THE CHECKLIST DAY 47

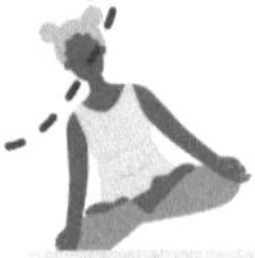

DID YOU MEDITATE?

HOW LONG?

HOW DO YOU FEEL?

DID YOU MAKE SURE TO BREATHE?

DON'T FORGET YOUR MANTRAS.

MEDS AND HERBS INTAKE

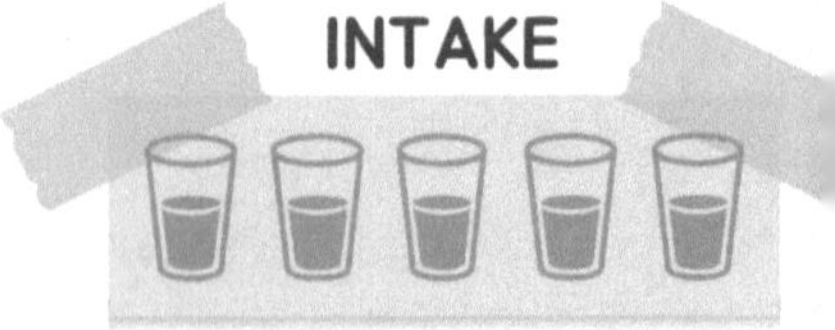

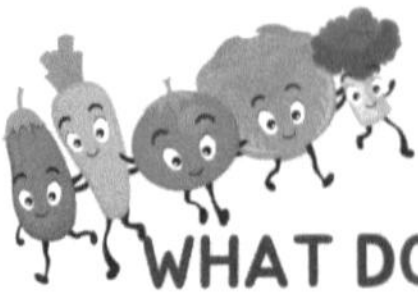

WHAT DOES YOUR MEAL LOOK LIKE TODAY

Breakfast:

Lunch:

Dinner:

Snack:

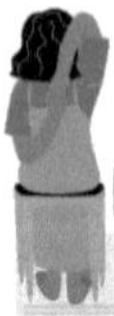

HOW WERE YOUR MOVEMENTS TODAY?

LETS GO THROUGH THE CHECKLIST DAY 48

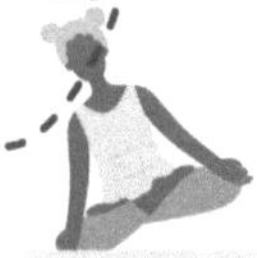

DID YOU MEDITATE?

HOW LONG?

HOW DO YOU FEEL?

DID YOU MAKE SURE TO BREATHE?

DON'T FORGET YOUR MANTRAS.

MEDS AND HERBS INTAKE

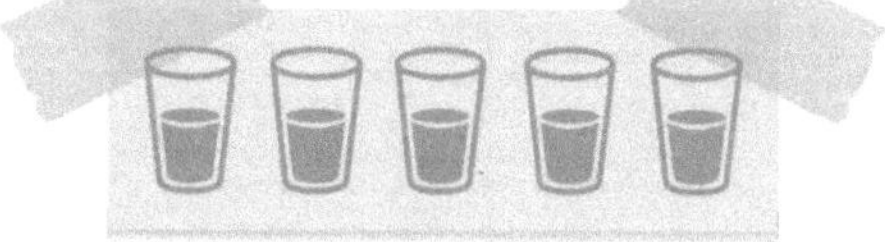

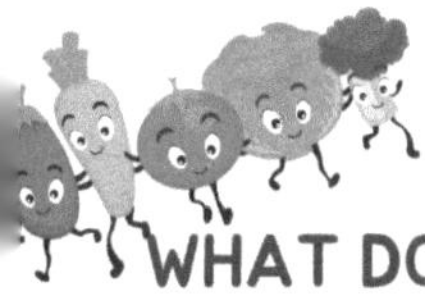

WHAT DOES YOUR MEAL LOOK LIKE TODAY

Breakfast:

Lunch:

Dinner:

Snack:

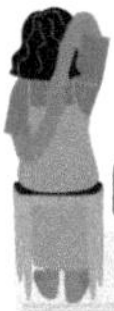

HOW WERE YOUR MOVEMENTS TODAY?

LETS GO THROUGH THE CHECKLIST

DAY 49

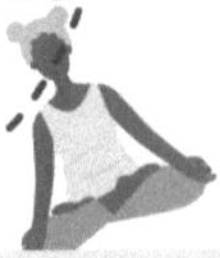

DID YOU MEDITATE?

HOW LONG?

HOW DO YOU FEEL?

DID YOU MAKE SURE TO BREATHE?

DON'T FORGET YOUR MANTRAS.

MEDS AND HERBS INTAKE

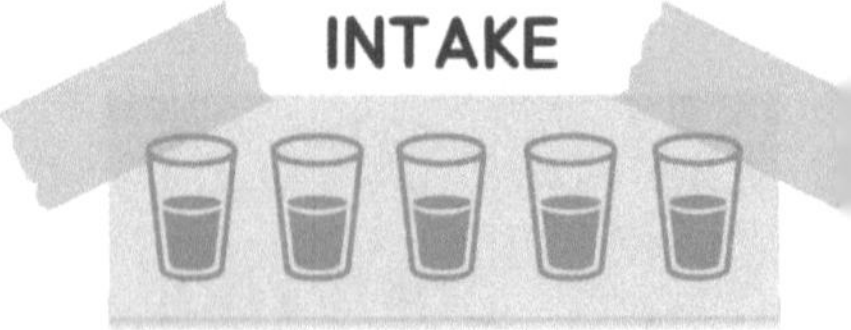

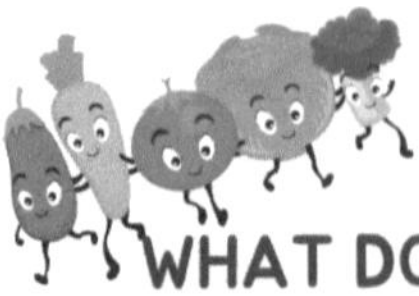

WHAT DOES YOUR MEAL LOOK LIKE TODAY

Breakfast:

Lunch:

Dinner:

Snack:

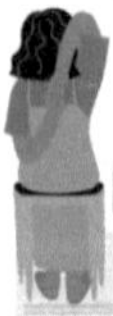

HOW WERE YOUR MOVEMENTS TODAY?

MAKE SURE TO MASSAGE THOSE BREASTS. IT HELPS WITH LOOSENING UP THE TISSUE AND IT HELPS WITH CIRCULATION FOR CORRECT HEALING. SUPER IMPORTANT! C'MON! LETS' GO!

LETS GO THROUGH THE CHECKLIST DAY 50

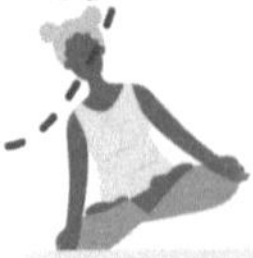

DID YOU MEDITATE?

HOW LONG?

HOW DO YOU FEEL?

DID YOU MAKE SURE TO BREATHE?

DON'T FORGET YOUR MANTRAS.

MEDS AND HERBS INTAKE

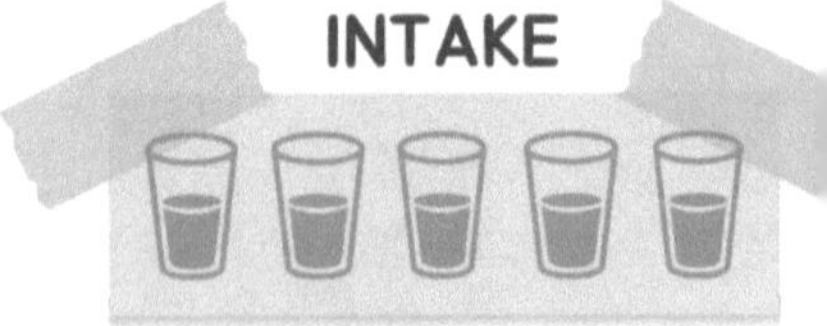

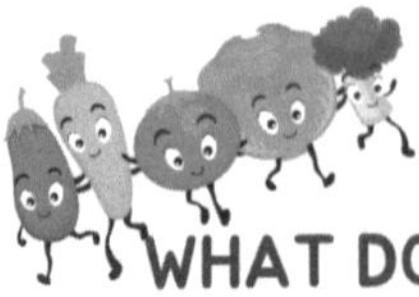

WHAT DOES YOUR MEAL LOOK LIKE TODAY

Breakfast:

Lunch:

Dinner:

Snack:

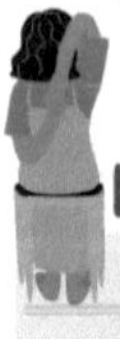

HOW WERE YOUR MOVEMENTS TODAY?

LETS GO THROUGH THE CHECKLIST DAY 51

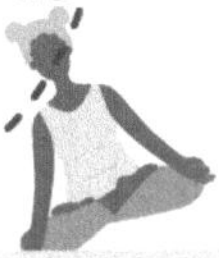

DID YOU MEDITATE?

HOW LONG?

HOW DO YOU FEEL?

DID YOU MAKE SURE TO BREATHE?

DON'T FORGET YOUR MANTRAS.

MEDS AND HERBS INTAKE

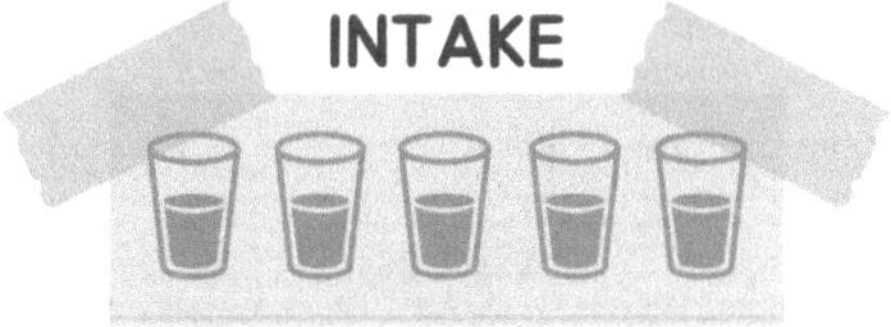

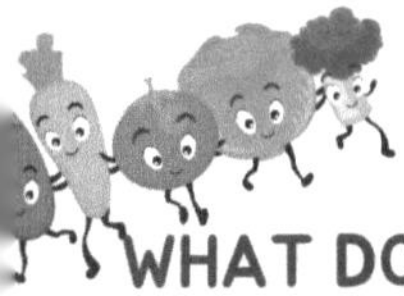

WHAT DOES YOUR MEAL LOOK LIKE TODAY

Breakfast:

Lunch:

Dinner:

Snack:

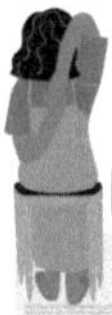

HOW WERE YOUR MOVEMENTS TODAY?

LETS GO THROUGH THE CHECKLIST DAY 52

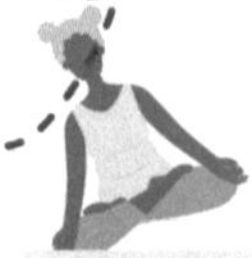

DID YOU MEDITATE?

HOW LONG?

HOW DO YOU FEEL?

DID YOU MAKE SURE TO BREATHE?

DON'T FORGET YOUR MANTRAS.

MEDS AND HERBS INTAKE

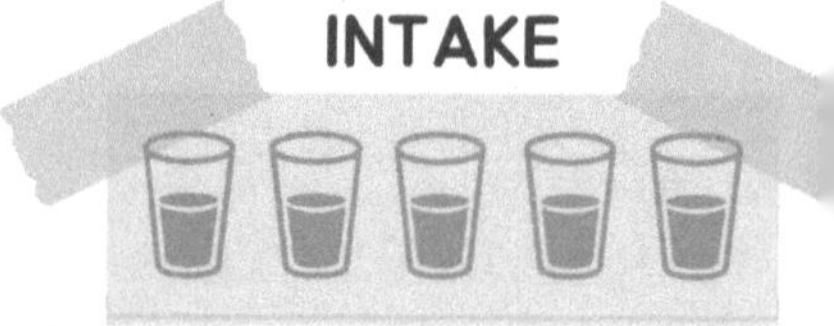

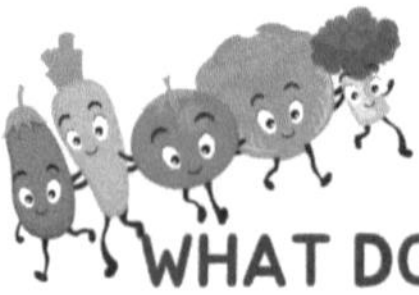

WHAT DOES YOUR MEAL LOOK LIKE TODAY

Breakfast:

Lunch:

Dinner:

Snack:

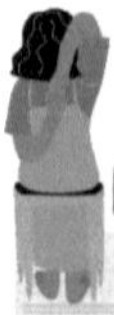

HOW WERE YOUR MOVEMENTS TODAY?

LETS GO THROUGH THE CHECKLIST DAY 53

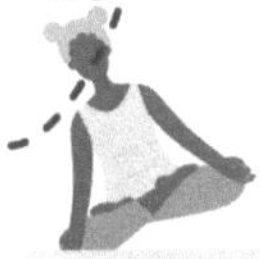

DID YOU MEDITATE?

HOW LONG?

HOW DO YOU FEEL?

DID YOU MAKE SURE TO BREATHE?

DON'T FORGET YOUR MANTRAS.

MEDS AND HERBS INTAKE

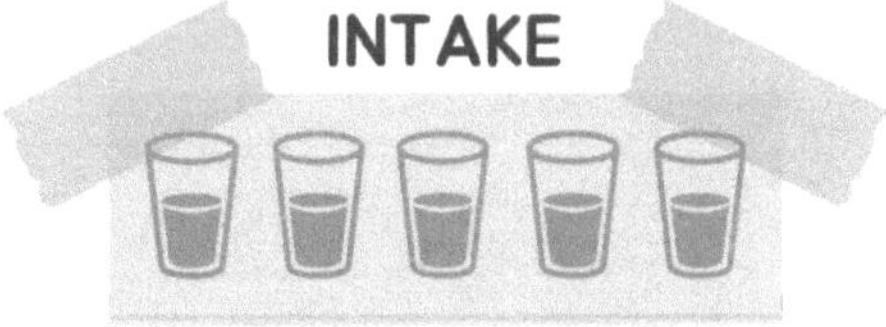

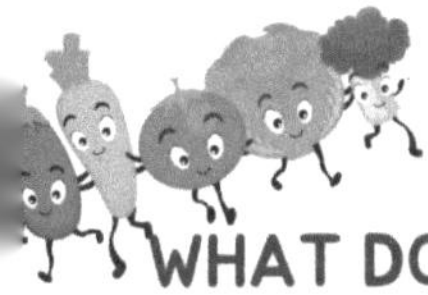

WHAT DOES YOUR MEAL LOOK LIKE TODAY

Breakfast:

Lunch:

Dinner:

Snack:

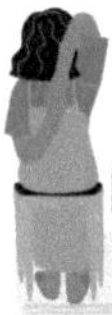

HOW WERE YOUR MOVEMENTS TODAY?

LETS GO THROUGH THE CHECKLIST DAY 54

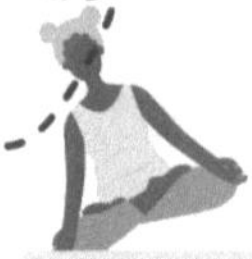

DID YOU MEDITATE?

HOW LONG?

HOW DO YOU FEEL?

DID YOU MAKE SURE TO BREATHE?

DON'T FORGET YOUR MANTRAS.

MEDS AND HERBS INTAKE

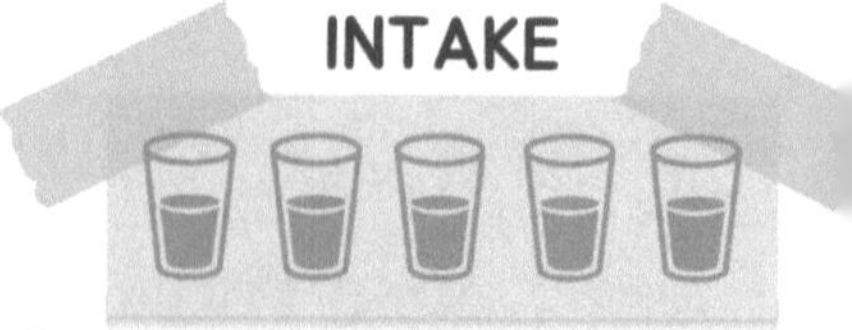

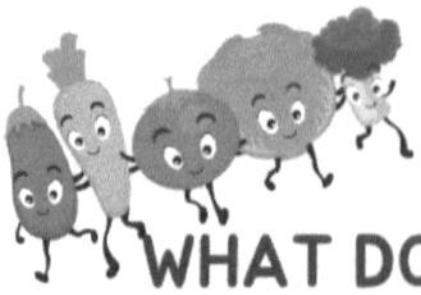

WHAT DOES YOUR MEAL LOOK LIKE TODAY

Breakfast:

Lunch:

Dinner:

Snack:

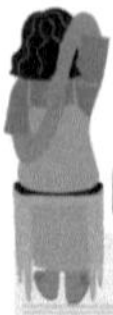

HOW WERE YOUR MOVEMENTS TODAY?

LETS GO THROUGH THE CHECKLIST DAY 55

DID YOU MEDITATE?

HOW LONG?

HOW DO YOU FEEL?

DID YOU MAKE SURE TO BREATHE?

DON'T FORGET YOUR MANTRAS.

MEDS AND HERBS INTAKE

WHAT DOES YOUR MEAL LOOK LIKE TODAY

Breakfast:

Lunch:

Dinner:

Snack:

HOW WERE YOUR MOVEMENTS TODAY?

LETS GO THROUGH THE CHECKLIST

DAY 56

DID YOU MEDITATE?

HOW LONG?

HOW DO YOU FEEL?

DID YOU MAKE SURE TO BREATHE?

DON'T FORGET YOUR MANTRAS.

MEDS AND HERBS INTAKE

WHAT DOES YOUR MEAL LOOK LIKE TODAY

Breakfast:

Lunch:

Dinner:

Snack:

HOW WERE YOUR MOVEMENTS TODAY?

REMEMBER SELF CARE!

LET SOMEONE ELSE COOK, CLEAN OR DO THE DISHES!

THIS IS ABOUT YOU.

CONTINUE TO TAKE CARE OF YOU!

LETS GO THROUGH THE CHECKLIST DAY 57

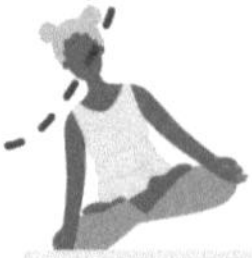

DID YOU MEDITATE?

HOW LONG?

HOW DO YOU FEEL?

DID YOU MAKE SURE TO BREATHE?

DON'T FORGET YOUR MANTRAS.

MEDS AND HERBS INTAKE

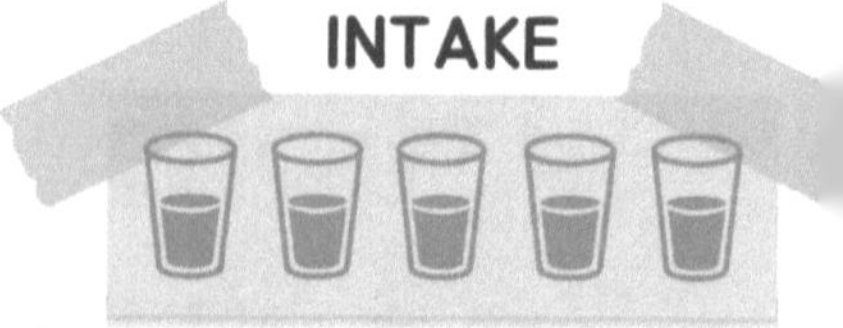

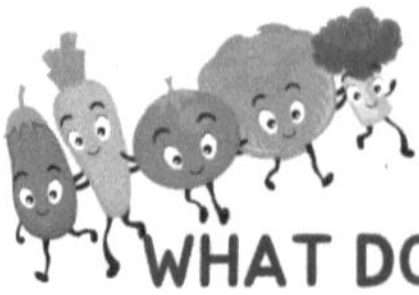

WHAT DOES YOUR MEAL LOOK LIKE TODAY

Breakfast:

Lunch:

Dinner:

Snack:

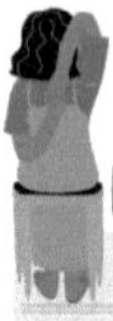

HOW WERE YOUR MOVEMENTS TODAY?

LETS GO THROUGH THE CHECKLIST DAY 58

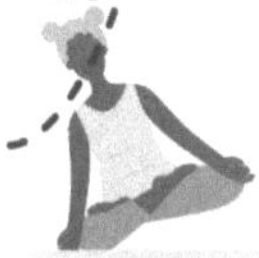

DID YOU MEDITATE?

HOW LONG?

HOW DO YOU FEEL?

DID YOU MAKE SURE TO BREATHE?

DON'T FORGET YOUR MANTRAS.

MEDS AND HERBS INTAKE

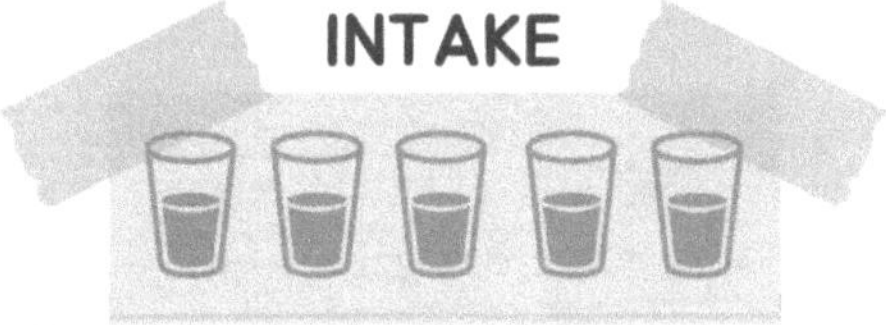

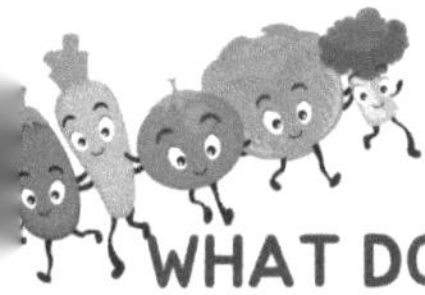

WHAT DOES YOUR MEAL LOOK LIKE TODAY

Breakfast:

Lunch:

Dinner:

Snack:

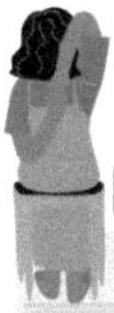

HOW WERE YOUR MOVEMENTS TODAY?

LETS GO THROUGH THE CHECKLIST
DAY 59

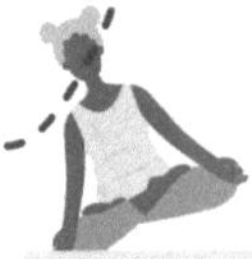

DID YOU MEDITATE?

HOW LONG?

HOW DO YOU FEEL?

DID YOU MAKE SURE TO BREATHE?

DON'T FORGET YOUR MANTRAS.

MEDS AND HERBS INTAKE

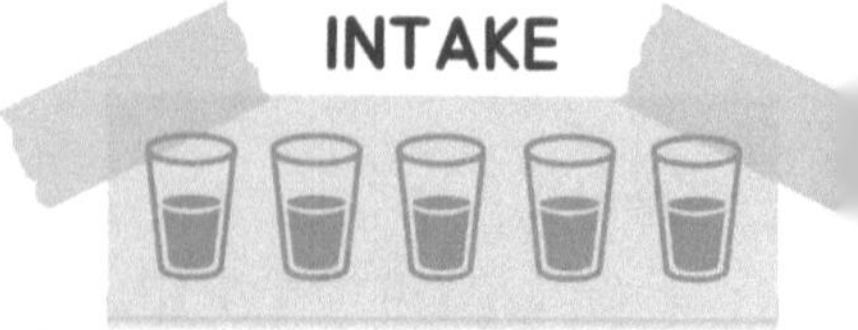

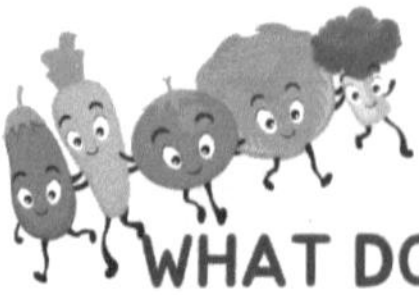

WHAT DOES YOUR MEAL LOOK LIKE TODAY

Breakfast:

Lunch:

Dinner:

Snack:

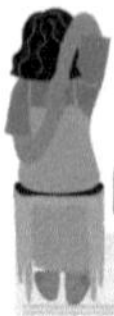

HOW WERE YOUR MOVEMENTS TODAY?

LETS GO THROUGH THE CHECKLIST DAY 60

DID YOU MEDITATE?

HOW LONG?

HOW DO YOU FEEL?

DID YOU MAKE SURE TO BREATHE?

DON'T FORGET YOUR MANTRAS.

MEDS AND HERBS INTAKE

WHAT DOES YOUR MEAL LOOK LIKE TODAY

Breakfast:

Lunch:

Dinner:

Snack:

HOW WERE YOUR MOVEMENTS TODAY?

LETS GO THROUGH THE CHECKLIST DAY 61

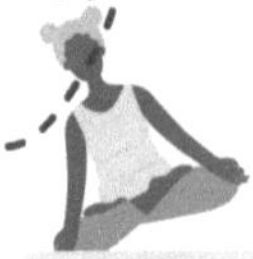

DID YOU MEDITATE?

HOW LONG?

HOW DO YOU FEEL?

DID YOU MAKE SURE TO BREATHE?

DON'T FORGET YOUR MANTRAS.

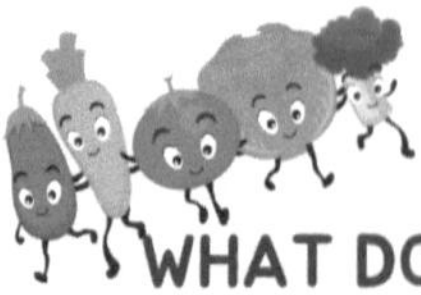

WHAT DOES YOUR MEAL LOOK LIKE TODAY

Breakfast:

Lunch:

Dinner:

Snack:

MEDS AND HERBS INTAKE

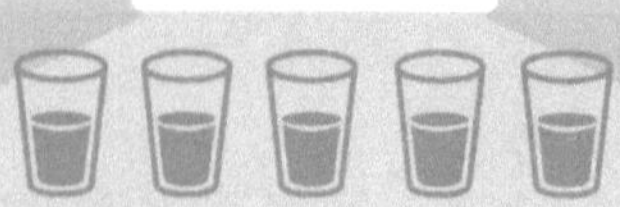

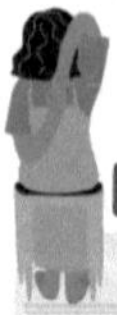

HOW WERE YOUR MOVEMENTS TODAY?

LETS GO THROUGH THE CHECKLIST

DAY 62

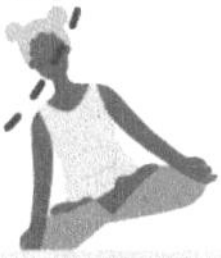

DID YOU MEDITATE?

HOW LONG?

HOW DO YOU FEEL?

DID YOU MAKE SURE TO BREATHE?

DON'T FORGET YOUR MANTRAS.

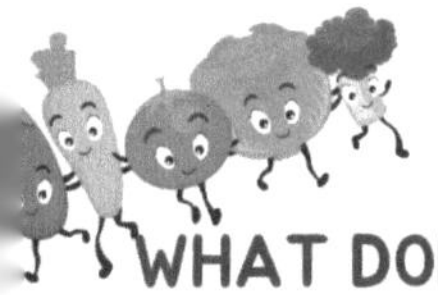

WHAT DOES YOUR MEAL LOOK LIKE TODAY

Breakfast:

Lunch:

Dinner:

Snack:

MEDS AND HERBS INTAKE

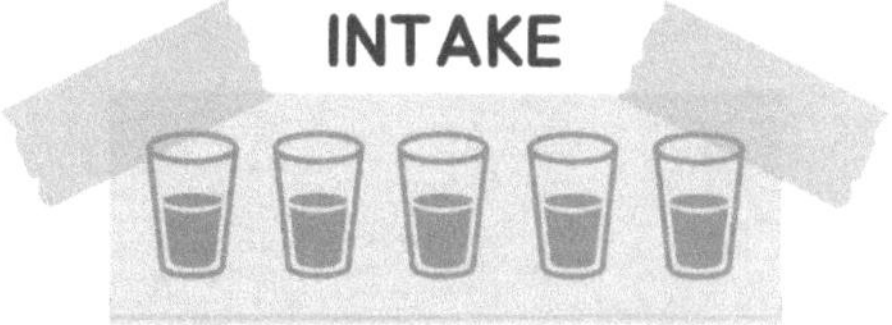

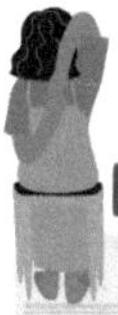

HOW WERE YOUR MOVEMENTS TODAY?

LETS GO THROUGH THE CHECKLIST DAY 63

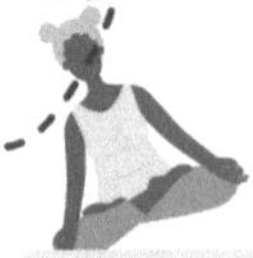

DID YOU MEDITATE?

HOW LONG?

HOW DO YOU FEEL?

DID YOU MAKE SURE TO BREATHE?

DON'T FORGET YOUR MANTRAS.

MEDS AND HERBS INTAKE

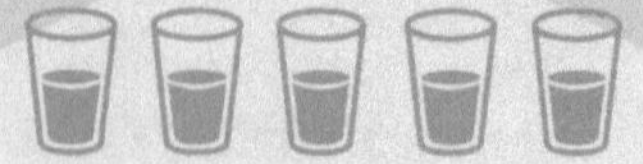

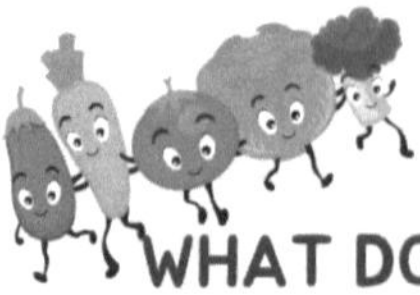

WHAT DOES YOUR MEAL LOOK LIKE TODAY

Breakfast:

Lunch:

Dinner:

Snack:

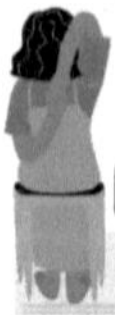

HOW WERE YOUR MOVEMENTS TODAY?

WHAT HAVE YOU
WORKED ON
BESIDES YOUR
HEALING?
I ENCOURAGE YOU
TO WORK ON A
PASSION OF YOURS,
IT WILL PROVIDE
PURPOSE!
THINK ABOUT IT
ATLEAST!

LETS GO THROUGH THE CHECKLIST DAY 64

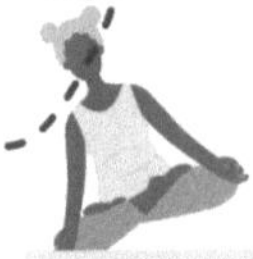

DID YOU MEDITATE?

HOW LONG?

HOW DO YOU FEEL?

DID YOU MAKE SURE TO BREATHE?

DON'T FORGET YOUR MANTRAS.

MEDS AND HERBS INTAKE

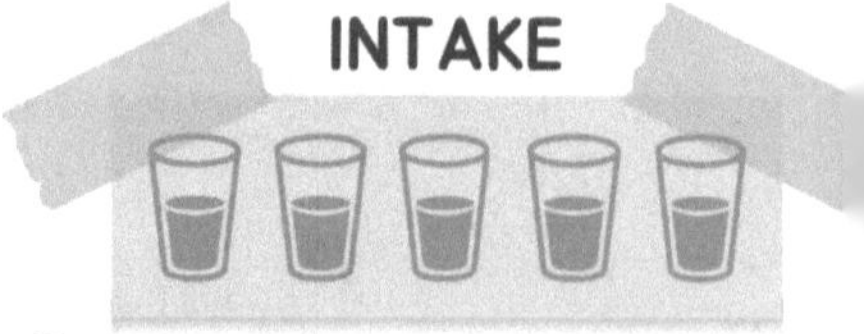

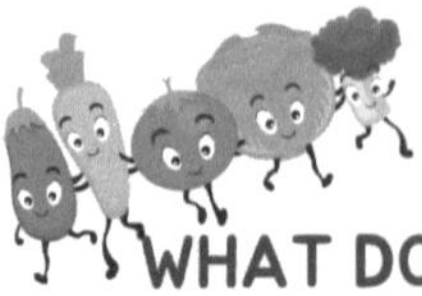

WHAT DOES YOUR MEAL LOOK LIKE TODAY

Breakfast:

Lunch:

Dinner:

Snack:

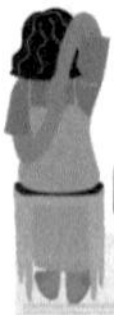

HOW WERE YOUR MOVEMENTS TODAY?

LETS GO THROUGH THE CHECKLIST DAY 65

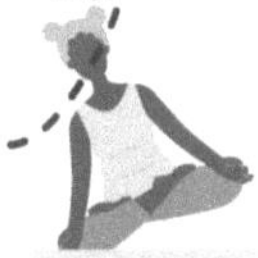

DID YOU MEDITATE?

HOW LONG?

HOW DO YOU FEEL?

DID YOU MAKE SURE TO BREATHE?

DON'T FORGET YOUR MANTRAS.

MEDS AND HERBS INTAKE

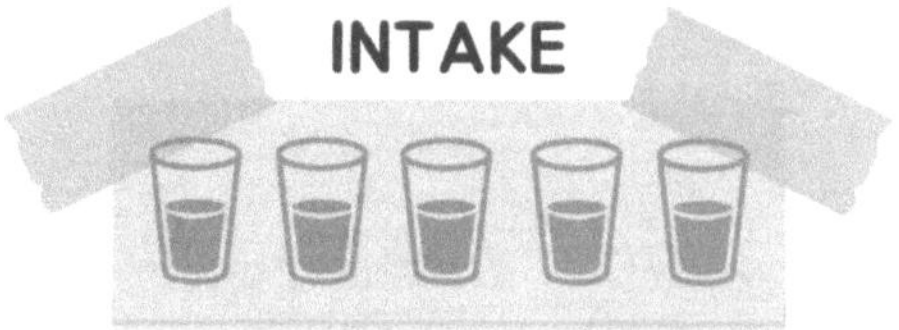

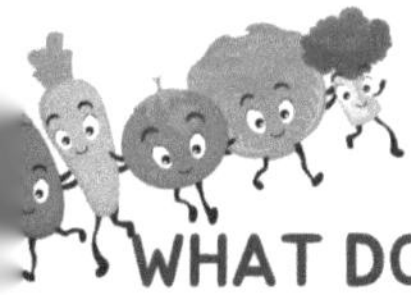

WHAT DOES YOUR MEAL LOOK LIKE TODAY

Breakfast:

Lunch:

Dinner:

Snack:

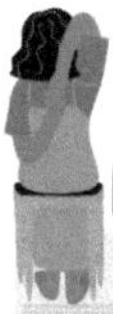

HOW WERE YOUR MOVEMENTS TODAY?

LETS GO THROUGH THE CHECKLIST DAY 66

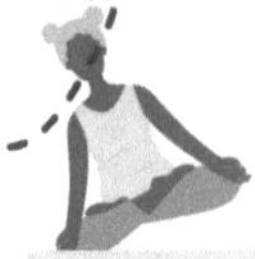

DID YOU MEDITATE?

HOW LONG?

HOW DO YOU FEEL?

DID YOU MAKE SURE TO BREATHE?

DON'T FORGET YOUR MANTRAS.

MEDS AND HERBS INTAKE

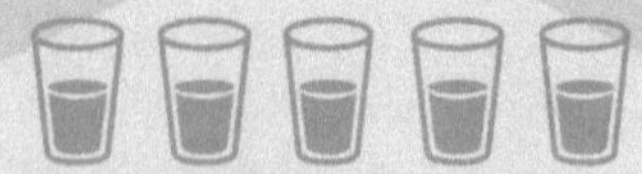

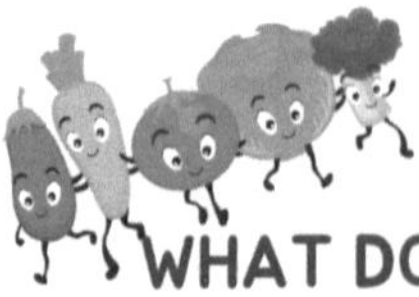

WHAT DOES YOUR MEAL LOOK LIKE TODAY

Breakfast:

Lunch:

Dinner:

Snack:

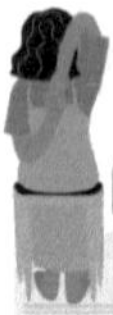

HOW WERE YOUR MOVEMENTS TODAY?

LETS GO THROUGH THE CHECKLIST DAY 67

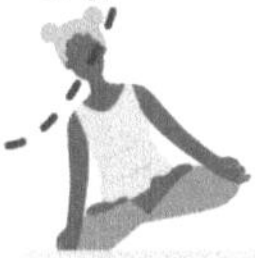

DID YOU MEDITATE?

HOW LONG?

HOW DO YOU FEEL?

DID YOU MAKE SURE TO BREATHE?

DON'T FORGET YOUR MANTRAS.

MEDS AND HERBS INTAKE

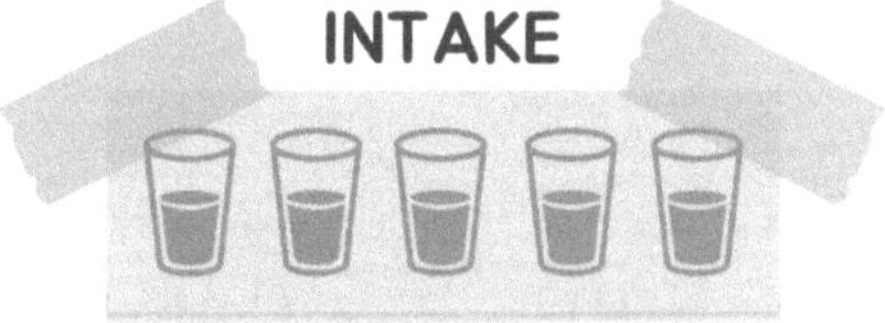

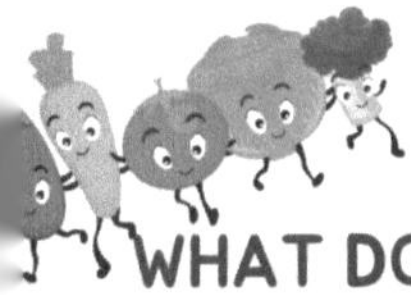

WHAT DOES YOUR MEAL LOOK LIKE TODAY

Breakfast:

Lunch:

Dinner:

Snack:

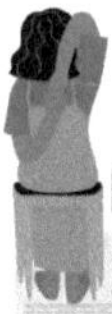

HOW WERE YOUR MOVEMENTS TODAY?

LETS GO THROUGH THE CHECKLIST DAY 68

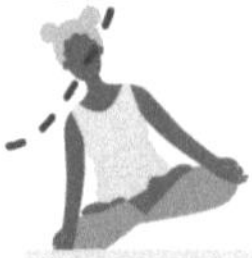

DID YOU MEDITATE?

HOW LONG?

HOW DO YOU FEEL?

DID YOU MAKE SURE TO BREATHE?

DON'T FORGET YOUR MANTRAS.

MEDS AND HERBS INTAKE

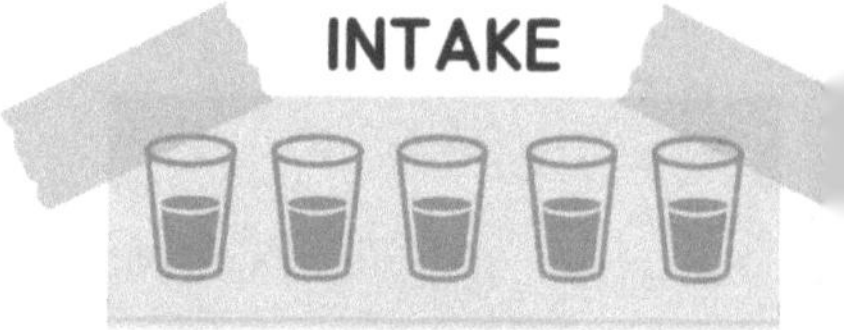

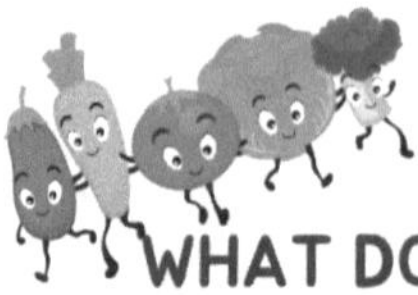

WHAT DOES YOUR MEAL LOOK LIKE TODAY

Breakfast:

Lunch:

Dinner:

Snack:

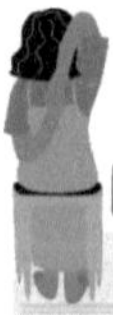

HOW WERE YOUR MOVEMENTS TODAY?

LETS GO THROUGH THE CHECKLIST DAY 69

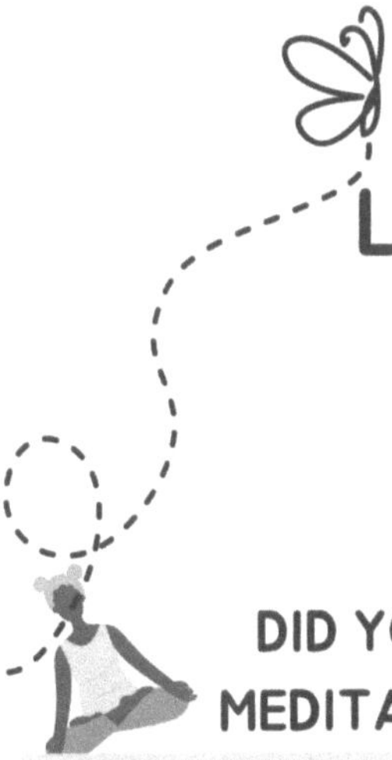

DID YOU MEDITATE?

HOW LONG?

HOW DO YOU FEEL?

DID YOU MAKE SURE TO BREATHE?

DON'T FORGET YOUR MANTRAS.

MEDS AND HERBS INTAKE

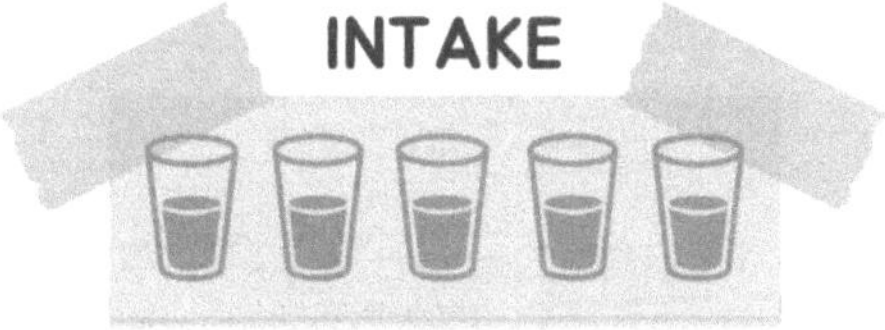

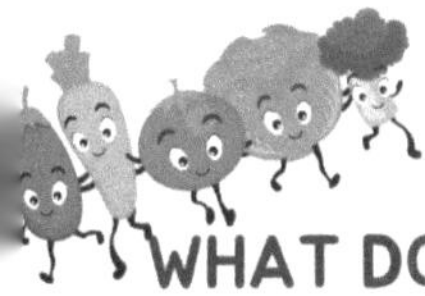

WHAT DOES YOUR MEAL LOOK LIKE TODAY

Breakfast:

Lunch:

Dinner:

Snack:

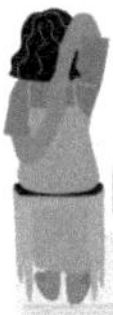

HOW WERE YOUR MOVEMENTS TODAY?

LETS GO THROUGH THE CHECKLIST DAY 70

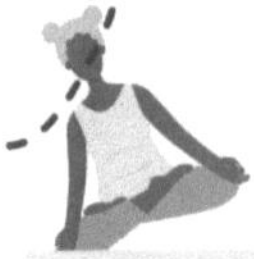

DID YOU MEDITATE?

HOW LONG?

HOW DO YOU FEEL?

DID YOU MAKE SURE TO BREATHE?

DON'T FORGET YOUR MANTRAS.

MEDS AND HERBS INTAKE

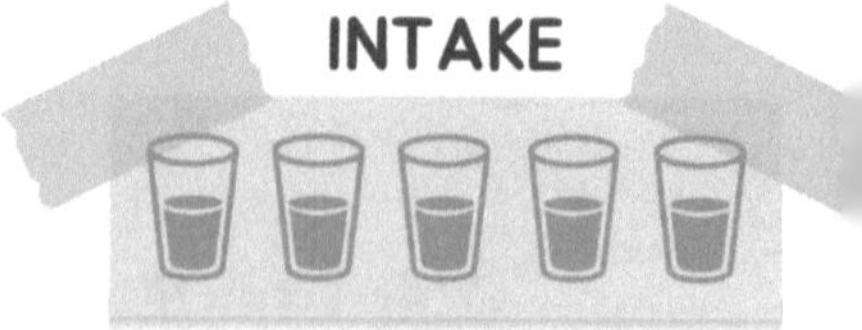

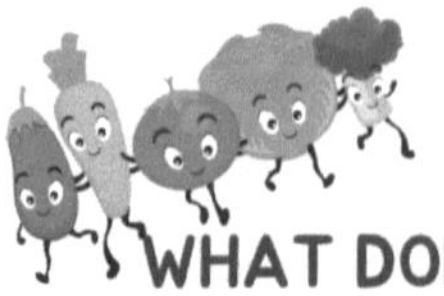

WHAT DOES YOUR MEAL LOOK LIKE TODAY

Breakfast:

Lunch:

Dinner:

Snack:

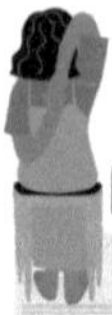

HOW WERE YOUR MOVEMENTS TODAY?

CAN YOU BELIEVE
YOU WENT THROUGH
70 DAYS OF
HEALING?
YOU HAVE GOTTEN
STRONGER
MENTALLY,
SPIRITUALLY,
EMOTIONALLY AND
PHYSICALLY EACH
DAY! LOOK AT YOU!

LETS GO THROUGH THE CHECKLIST DAY 71

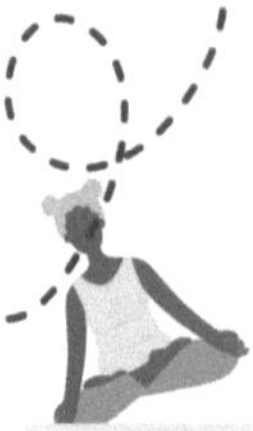

DID YOU MEDITATE?

HOW LONG?

HOW DO YOU FEEL?

DID YOU MAKE SURE TO BREATHE?

DON'T FORGET YOUR MANTRAS.

MEDS AND HERBS INTAKE

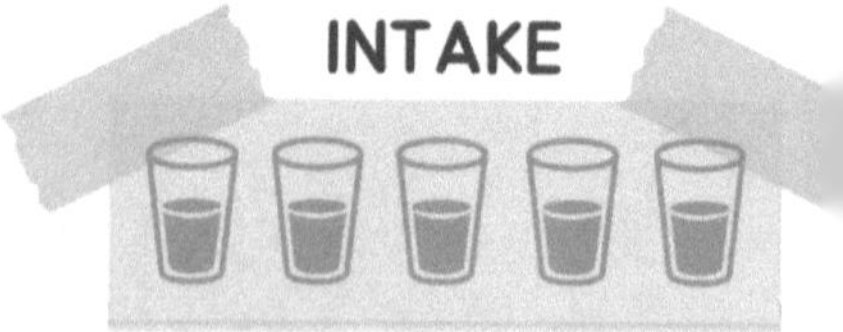

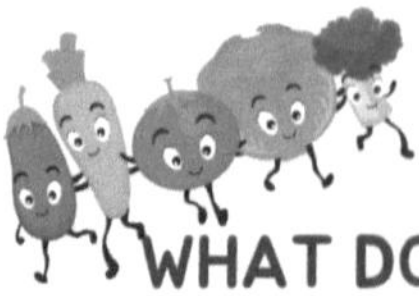

WHAT DOES YOUR MEAL LOOK LIKE TODAY

Breakfast:

Lunch:

Dinner:

Snack:

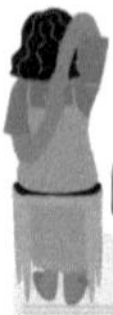

HOW WERE YOUR MOVEMENTS TODAY?

LETS GO THROUGH THE CHECKLIST
DAY 72

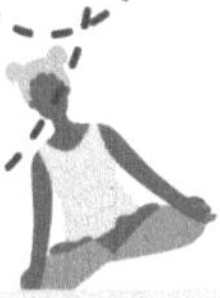

DID YOU MEDITATE?

HOW LONG?

HOW DO YOU FEEL?

DID YOU MAKE SURE TO BREATHE?

DON'T FORGET YOUR MANTRAS.

MEDS AND HERBS INTAKE

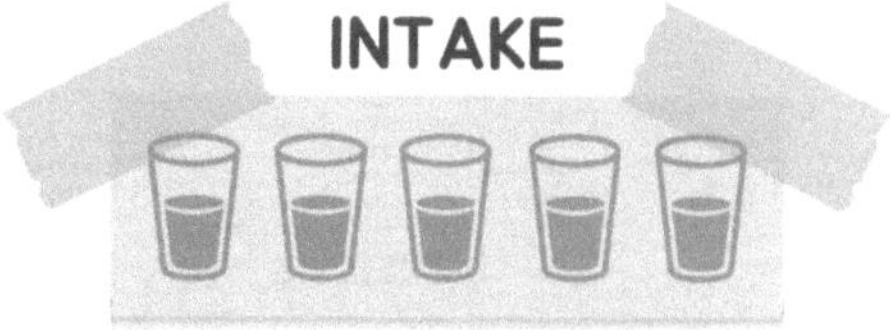

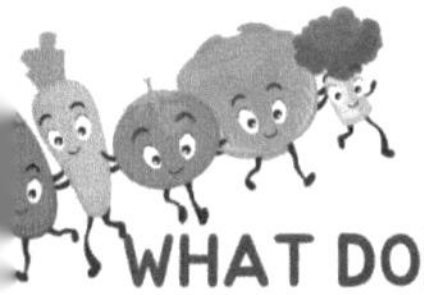

WHAT DOES YOUR MEAL LOOK LIKE TODAY

Breakfast:

Lunch:

Dinner:

Snack:

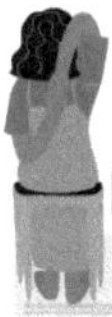

HOW WERE YOUR MOVEMENTS TODAY?

LETS GO THROUGH THE CHECKLIST
DAY 73

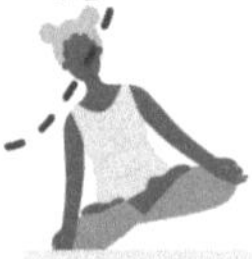

DID YOU MEDITATE?

HOW LONG?

HOW DO YOU FEEL?

DID YOU MAKE SURE TO BREATHE?

DON'T FORGET YOUR MANTRAS.

MEDS AND HERBS INTAKE

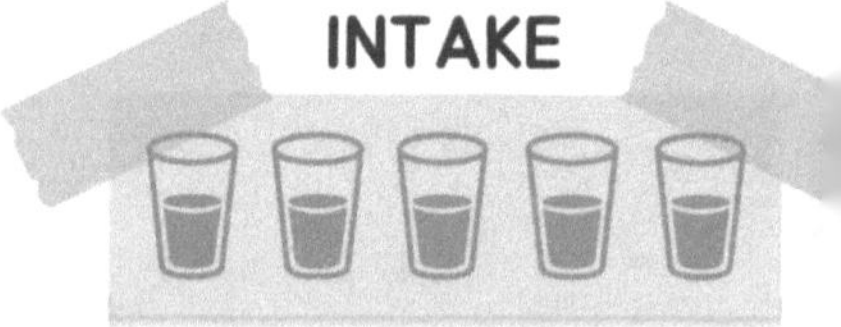

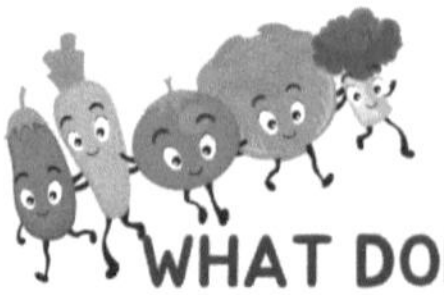

WHAT DOES YOUR MEAL LOOK LIKE TODAY

Breakfast:

Lunch:

Dinner:

Snack:

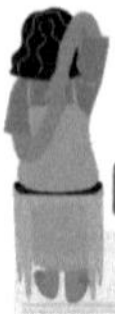

HOW WERE YOUR MOVEMENTS TODAY?

LETS GO THROUGH THE CHECKLIST DAY 74

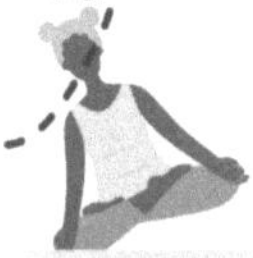

DID YOU MEDITATE?

HOW LONG?

HOW DO YOU FEEL?

DID YOU MAKE SURE TO BREATHE?

DON'T FORGET YOUR MANTRAS.

MEDS AND HERBS INTAKE

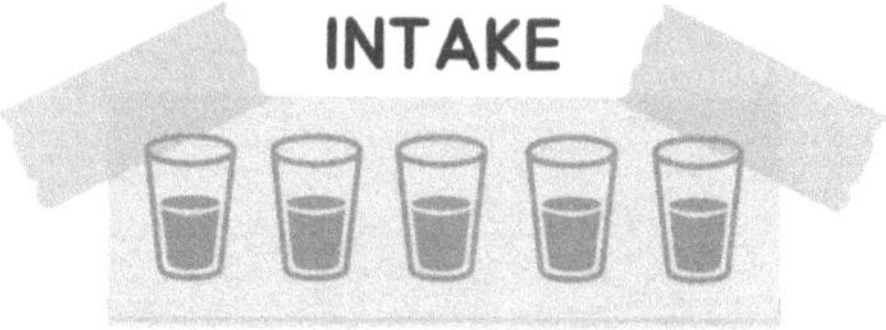

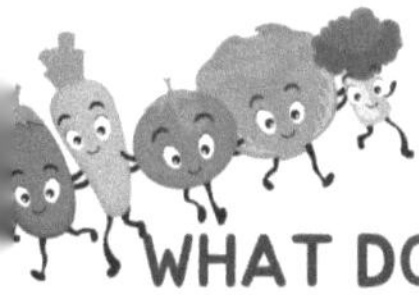

WHAT DOES YOUR MEAL LOOK LIKE TODAY

Breakfast:

Lunch:

Dinner:

Snack:

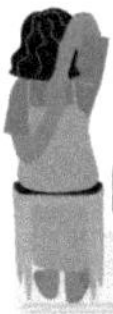

HOW WERE YOUR MOVEMENTS TODAY?

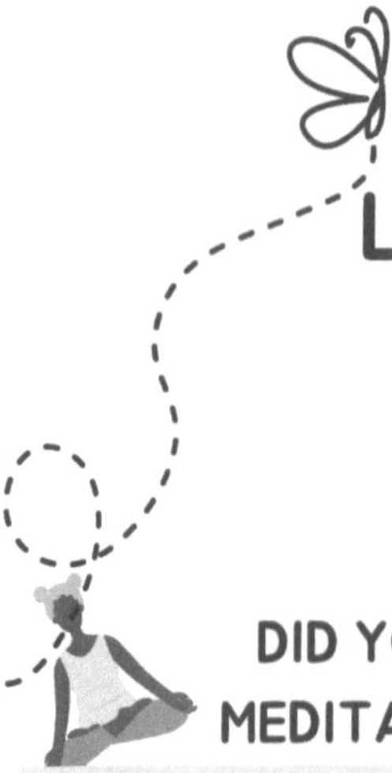

LETS GO THROUGH THE CHECKLIST DAY 75

DID YOU MEDITATE?

HOW LONG?

HOW DO YOU FEEL?

DID YOU MAKE SURE TO BREATHE?

DON'T FORGET YOUR MANTRAS.

MEDS AND HERBS INTAKE

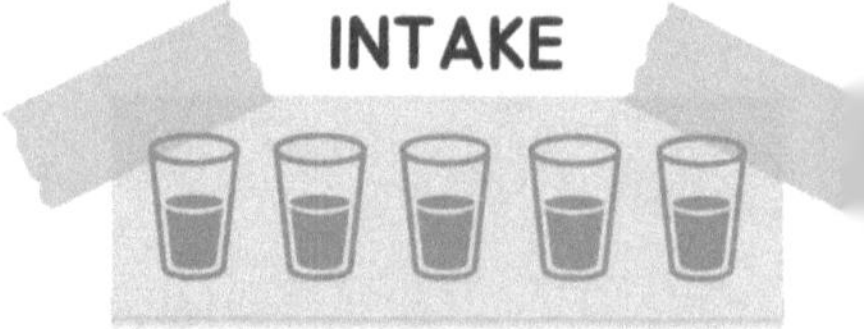

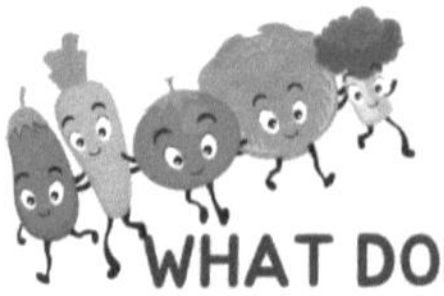

WHAT DOES YOUR MEAL LOOK LIKE TODAY

Breakfast:

Lunch:

Dinner:

Snack:

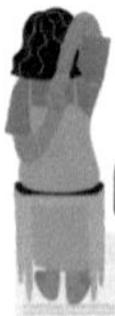

HOW WERE YOUR MOVEMENTS TODAY?

LETS GO THROUGH THE CHECKLIST DAY 76

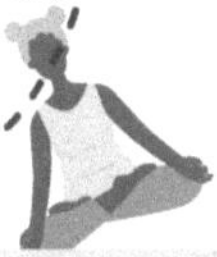

DID YOU MEDITATE?

HOW LONG?

HOW DO YOU FEEL?

DID YOU MAKE SURE TO BREATHE?

DON'T FORGET YOUR MANTRAS.

MEDS AND HERBS INTAKE

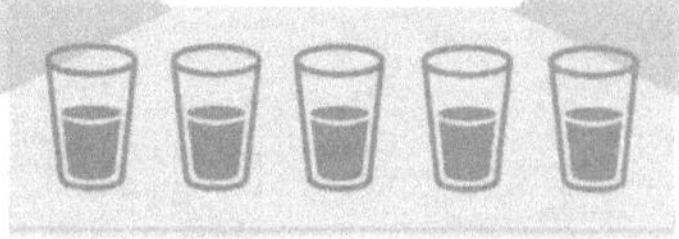

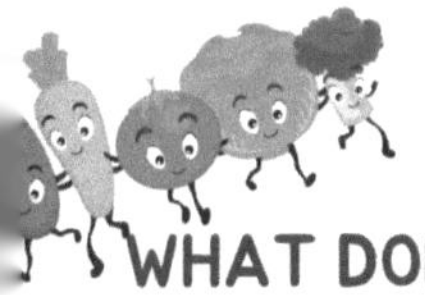

WHAT DOES YOUR MEAL LOOK LIKE TODAY

Breakfast:

Lunch:

Dinner:

Snack:

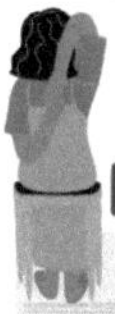

HOW WERE YOUR MOVEMENTS TODAY?

LETS GO THROUGH THE CHECKLIST
DAY 77

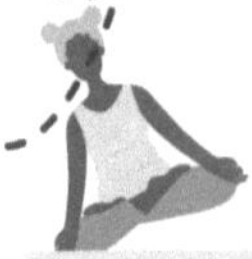

DID YOU MEDITATE?

HOW LONG?

HOW DO YOU FEEL?

DID YOU MAKE SURE TO BREATHE?

DON'T FORGET YOUR MANTRAS.

MEDS AND HERBS INTAKE

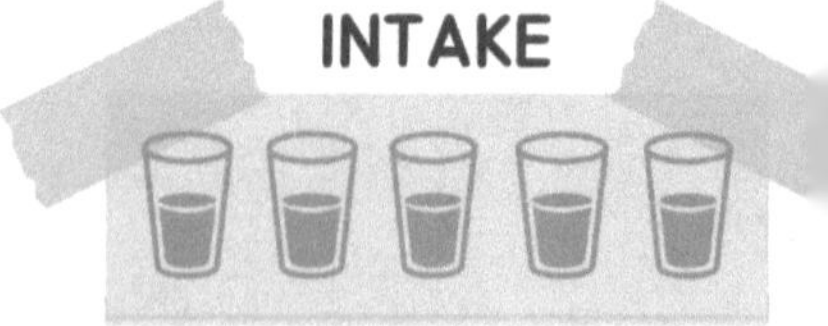

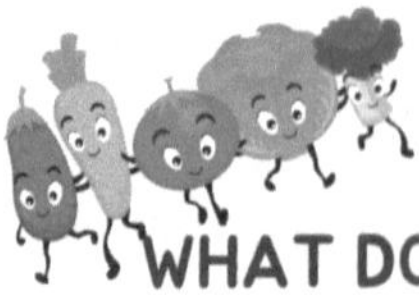

WHAT DOES YOUR MEAL LOOK LIKE TODAY

Breakfast:

Lunch:

Dinner:

Snack:

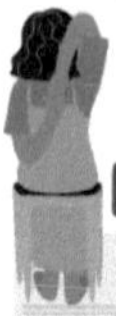

HOW WERE YOUR MOVEMENTS TODAY?

I AM HOPING YOU HAVEN'T HAD ANY COMPLICATIONS TO PROLONG THE PROCESS. IT MAY FEEL DISOURAGING SO I AM SENDING YOU LOVE EITHER WAY AND WISHING YOU A SUCCESSFUL JOURNEY

LETS GO THROUGH THE CHECKLIST

DAY 78

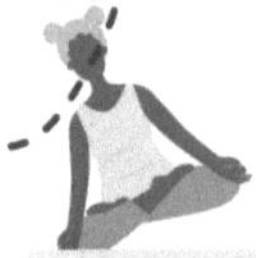

DID YOU MEDITATE?

HOW LONG?

HOW DO YOU FEEL?

DID YOU MAKE SURE TO BREATHE?

DON'T FORGET YOUR MANTRAS.

MEDS AND HERBS INTAKE

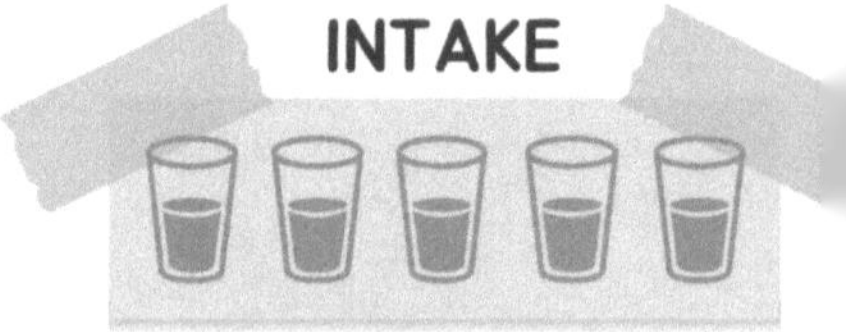

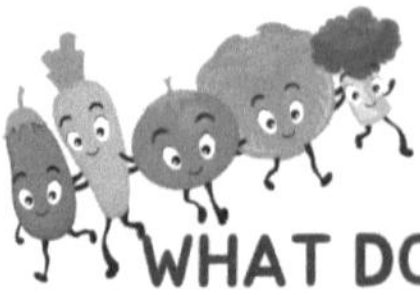

WHAT DOES YOUR MEAL LOOK LIKE TODAY

Breakfast:

Lunch:

Dinner:

Snack:

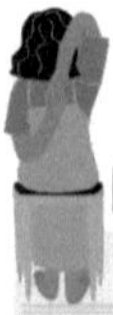

HOW WERE YOUR MOVEMENTS TODAY?

LETS GO THROUGH THE CHECKLIST

DAY 79

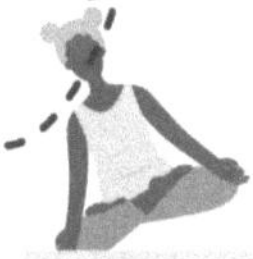

DID YOU MEDITATE?

HOW LONG?

HOW DO YOU FEEL?

DID YOU MAKE SURE TO BREATHE?

DON'T FORGET YOUR MANTRAS.

MEDS AND HERBS INTAKE

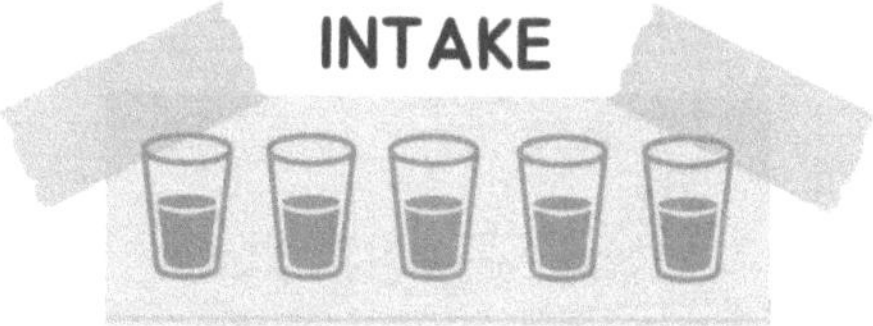

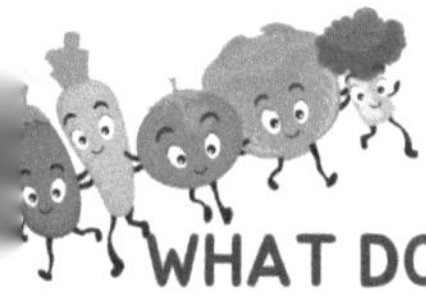

WHAT DOES YOUR MEAL LOOK LIKE TODAY

Breakfast:

Lunch:

Dinner:

Snack:

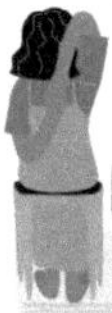

HOW WERE YOUR MOVEMENTS TODAY?

LETS GO THROUGH THE CHECKLIST DAY 80

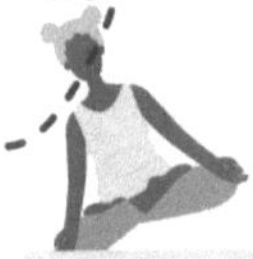

DID YOU MEDITATE?

HOW LONG?

HOW DO YOU FEEL?

DID YOU MAKE SURE TO BREATHE?

DON'T FORGET YOUR MANTRAS.

MEDS AND HERBS INTAKE

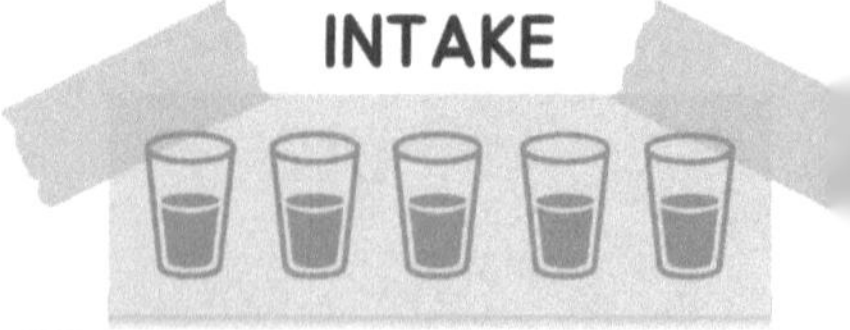

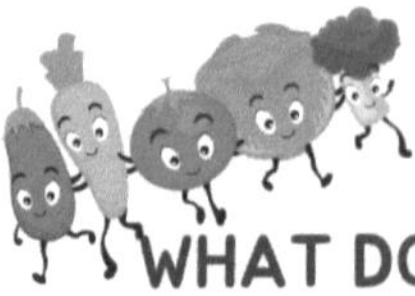

WHAT DOES YOUR MEAL LOOK LIKE TODAY

Breakfast:

Lunch:

Dinner:

Snack:

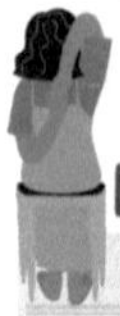

HOW WERE YOUR MOVEMENTS TODAY?

LETS GO THROUGH THE CHECKLIST DAY 81

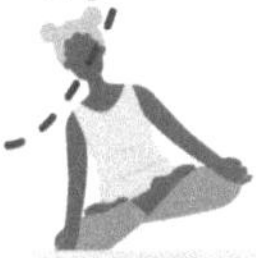

DID YOU MEDITATE?

HOW LONG?

HOW DO YOU FEEL?

DID YOU MAKE SURE TO BREATHE?

DON'T FORGET YOUR MANTRAS.

MEDS AND HERBS INTAKE

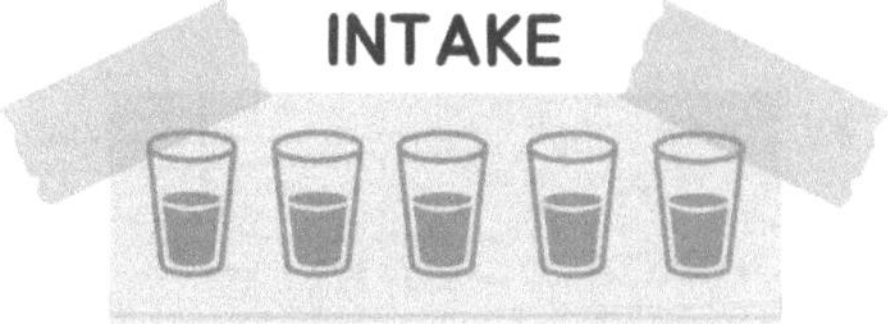

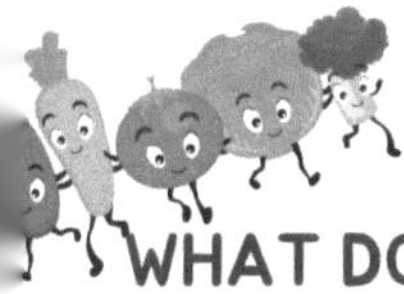

WHAT DOES YOUR MEAL LOOK LIKE TODAY

Breakfast:

Lunch:

Dinner:

Snack:

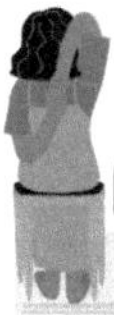

HOW WERE YOUR MOVEMENTS TODAY?

LETS GO THROUGH THE CHECKLIST DAY 82

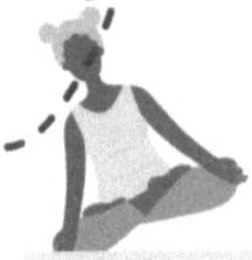

DID YOU MEDITATE?

HOW LONG?

HOW DO YOU FEEL?

DID YOU MAKE SURE TO BREATHE?

DON'T FORGET YOUR MANTRAS.

MEDS AND HERBS INTAKE

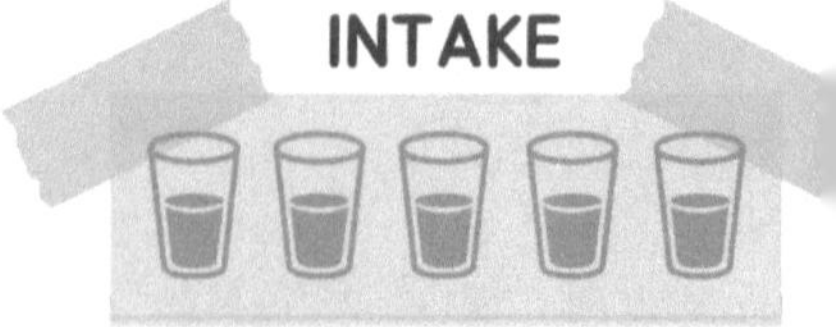

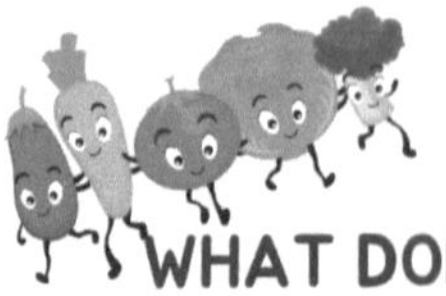

WHAT DOES YOUR MEAL LOOK LIKE TODAY

Breakfast:

Lunch:

Dinner:

Snack:

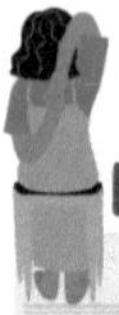

HOW WERE YOUR MOVEMENTS TODAY?

LETS GO THROUGH THE CHECKLIST DAY 83

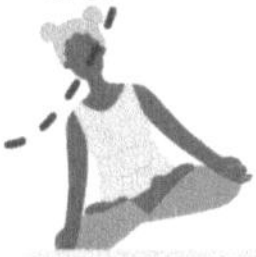

DID YOU MEDITATE?

HOW LONG?

HOW DO YOU FEEL?

DID YOU MAKE SURE TO BREATHE?

DON'T FORGET YOUR MANTRAS.

MEDS AND HERBS INTAKE

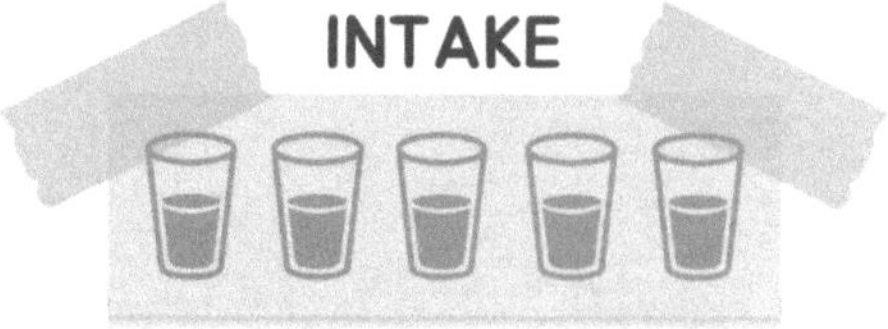

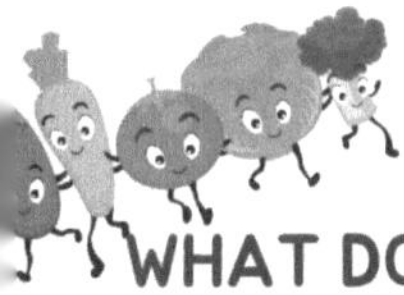

WHAT DOES YOUR MEAL LOOK LIKE TODAY

Breakfast:

Lunch:

Dinner:

Snack:

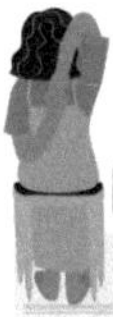

HOW WERE YOUR MOVEMENTS TODAY?

LETS GO THROUGH THE CHECKLIST DAY 84

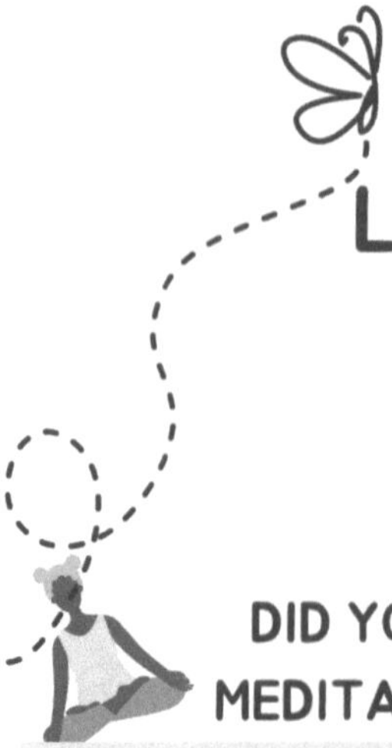

DID YOU MEDITATE?

HOW LONG?

HOW DO YOU FEEL?

DID YOU MAKE SURE TO BREATHE?

DON'T FORGET YOUR MANTRAS.

MEDS AND HERBS INTAKE

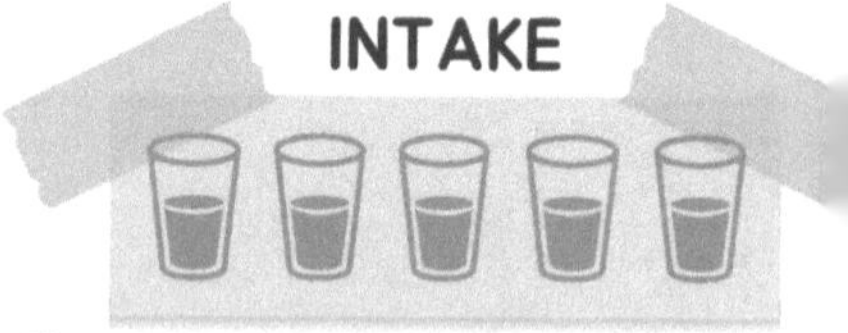

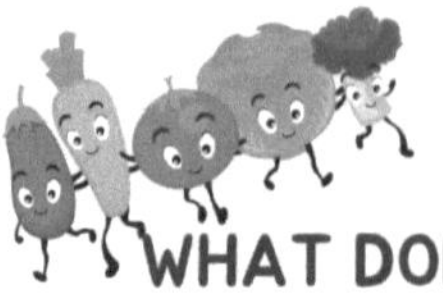

WHAT DOES YOUR MEAL LOOK LIKE TODAY

Breakfast:

Lunch:

Dinner:

Snack:

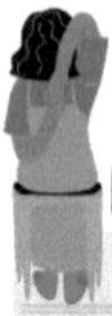

HOW WERE YOUR MOVEMENTS TODAY?

YOU ARE ALMOST AT THE 90 DAY MARK. HOW DO YOU FEEL? CAN YOU WALK WITHOUT HOLDING YOUR CHEST? CAN YOU PUT YOUR ARMS UP? CAN YOU LAUGH WITHOUT PAIN? BE PROUD AND REMEMBER IT IS STILL A PROCESS.

LETS GO THROUGH THE CHECKLIST DAY 85

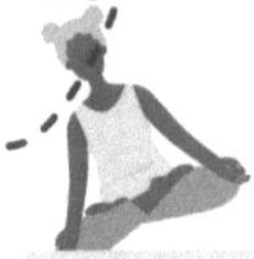

DID YOU MEDITATE?

HOW LONG?

HOW DO YOU FEEL?

DID YOU MAKE SURE TO BREATHE?

DON'T FORGET YOUR MANTRAS.

MEDS AND HERBS INTAKE

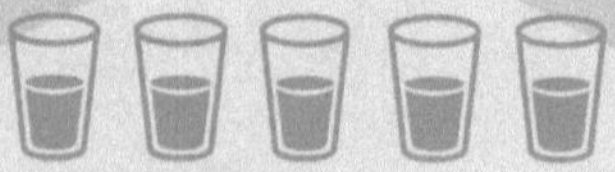

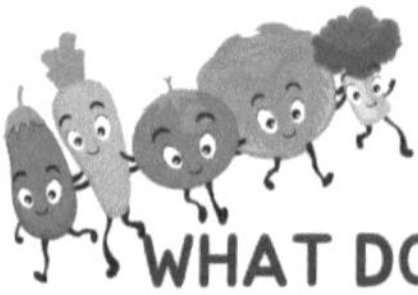

WHAT DOES YOUR MEAL LOOK LIKE TODAY

Breakfast:

Lunch:

Dinner:

Snack:

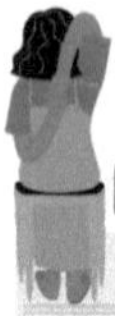

HOW WERE YOUR MOVEMENTS TODAY?

LETS GO THROUGH THE CHECKLIST DAY 86

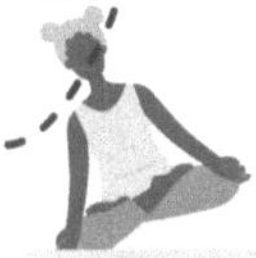

DID YOU MEDITATE?

HOW LONG?

HOW DO YOU FEEL?

DID YOU MAKE SURE TO BREATHE?

DON'T FORGET YOUR MANTRAS.

MEDS AND HERBS INTAKE

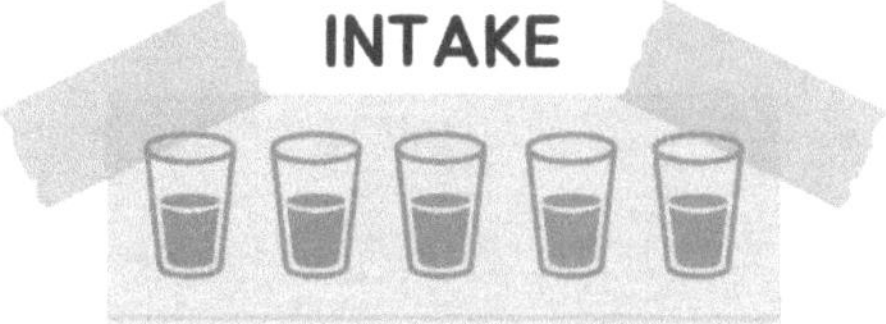

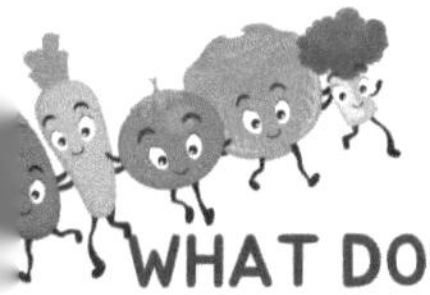

WHAT DOES YOUR MEAL LOOK LIKE TODAY

Breakfast:

Lunch:

Dinner:

Snack:

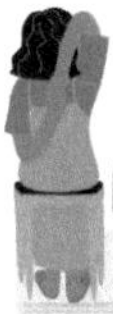

HOW WERE YOUR MOVEMENTS TODAY?

LETS GO THROUGH THE CHECKLIST DAY 87

DID YOU MEDITATE?

HOW LONG?

HOW DO YOU FEEL?

DID YOU MAKE SURE TO BREATHE?

DON'T FORGET YOUR MANTRAS.

MEDS AND HERBS INTAKE

WHAT DOES YOUR MEAL LOOK LIKE TODAY

Breakfast:

Lunch:

Dinner:

Snack:

HOW WERE YOUR MOVEMENTS TODAY?

LETS GO THROUGH THE CHECKLIST

DAY 88

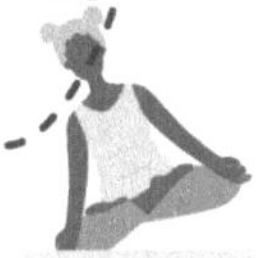

DID YOU MEDITATE?

HOW LONG?

HOW DO YOU FEEL?

DID YOU MAKE SURE TO BREATHE?

DON'T FORGET YOUR MANTRAS.

MEDS AND HERBS INTAKE

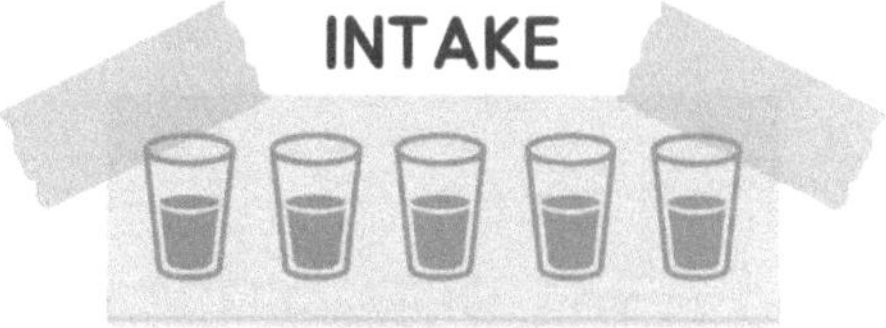

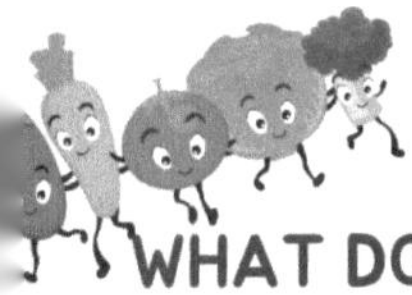

WHAT DOES YOUR MEAL LOOK LIKE TODAY

Breakfast:

Lunch:

Dinner:

Snack:

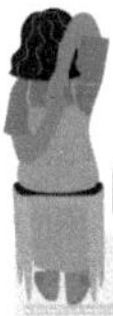

HOW WERE YOUR MOVEMENTS TODAY?

LETS GO THROUGH THE CHECKLIST DAY 89

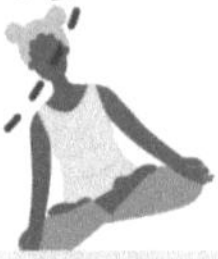

DID YOU MEDITATE?

HOW LONG?

HOW DO YOU FEEL?

DID YOU MAKE SURE TO BREATHE?

DON'T FORGET YOUR MANTRAS.

MEDS AND HERBS INTAKE

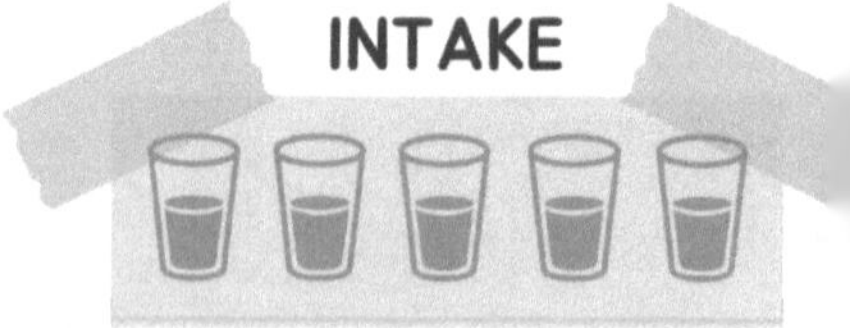

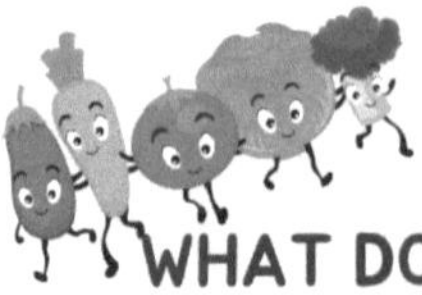

WHAT DOES YOUR MEAL LOOK LIKE TODAY

Breakfast:

Lunch:

Dinner:

Snack:

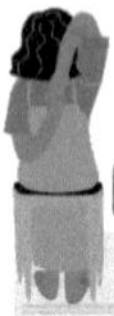

HOW WERE YOUR MOVEMENTS TODAY?

LETS GO THROUGH THE CHECKLIST DAY 90

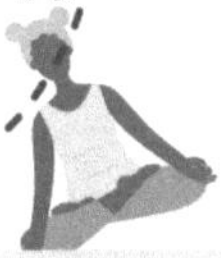

DID YOU MEDITATE?

HOW LONG?

HOW DO YOU FEEL?

DID YOU MAKE SURE TO BREATHE?

DON'T FORGET YOUR MANTRAS.

MEDS AND HERBS INTAKE

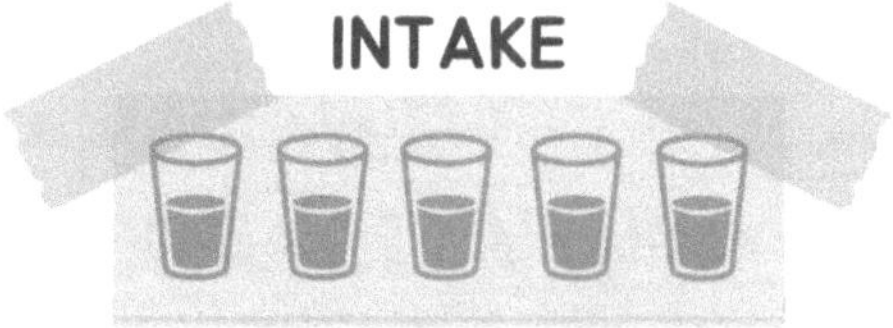

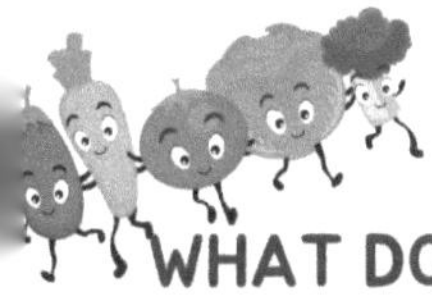

WHAT DOES YOUR MEAL LOOK LIKE TODAY

Breakfast:

Lunch:

Dinner:

Snack:

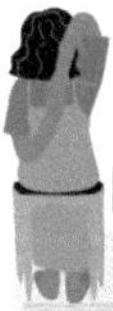

HOW WERE YOUR MOVEMENTS TODAY?

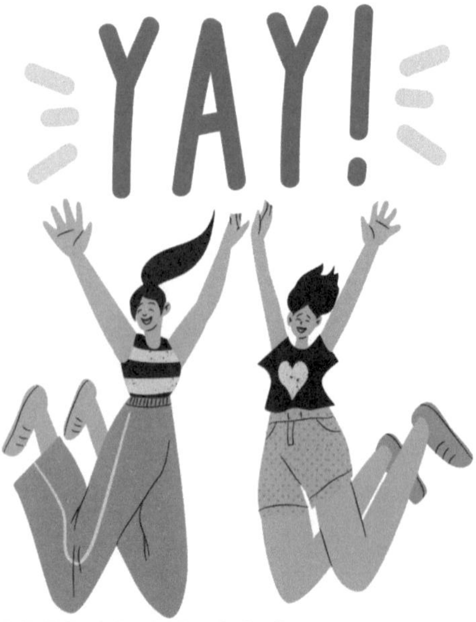

YOU COMPLETED YOUR 90 DAYS OF HEALING. THE JOURNEY IS NOT OVER. AS A MATTER OF FACT YOU ARE JUST BEGINNING. I ENCOURAGE YOU TO STILL PRACTICE THE 5 M'S

AS THE BODY IS STILL VERY MUCH GOING THROUGH A HEALING PROCESS.

YOU MAY READ OR HEAR THAT RECOVERY IS 6 TO 8 WEEKS BUT IT IS MUCH MORE THAN THAT.

EVEN WHEN YOU ARE FEELING BETTER, YOU MAY STILL HAVE MOMENTS OF DISCOMFORT AND PAIN MONTHS AFTER. SO BE CAREFUL, STAY HYDRATED, EAT WELL, MEDITATE, TAKE MEDS/HERBS AND BE SURE TO STAY ACTIVE AND MOVE.

Thank you for trusting
The GoodLook In Books to help
you during a very difficult time
in your life. You would see that
we focus on healing of all types,
from poetry form, to physical,
mental and spiritual. We like to
feel that after reading our
books that it provides a
positive outlook, clarity and a
sense of relief for your daily
lives.
We greatly appreciate you!

THE GOODLOOK IN BOOKS CORP

Made in United States
Troutdale, OR
06/19/2023

10682270R10070